Diverticular Disease of the Colon - Recent Knowledge of Physiopathology, Endoscopic Approaches, Clinical and Surgical Treatments

Edited by José Joaquim Ribeiro da Rocha and Marley Ribeiro Feitosa

Published in London, United Kingdom

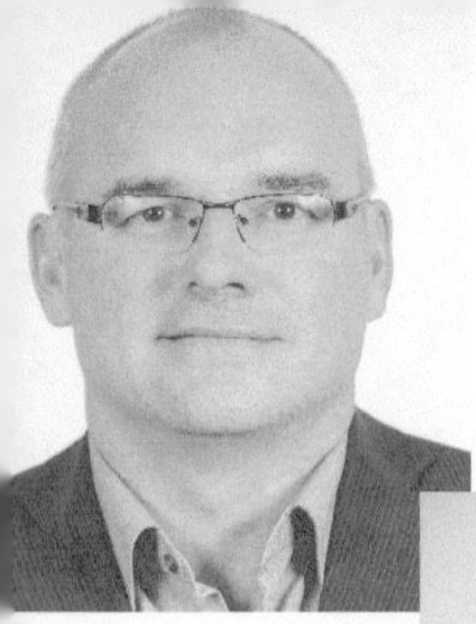

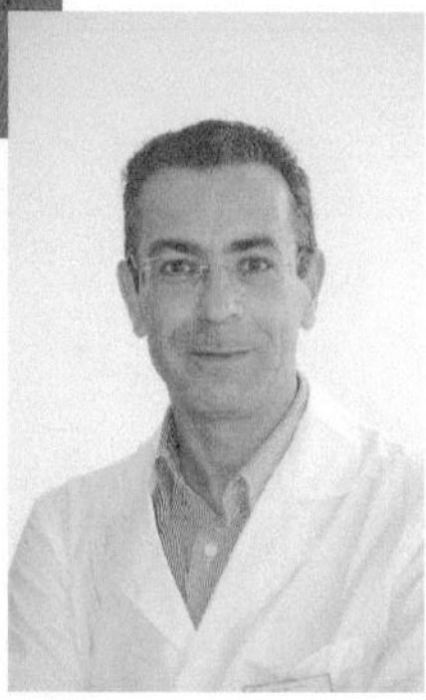

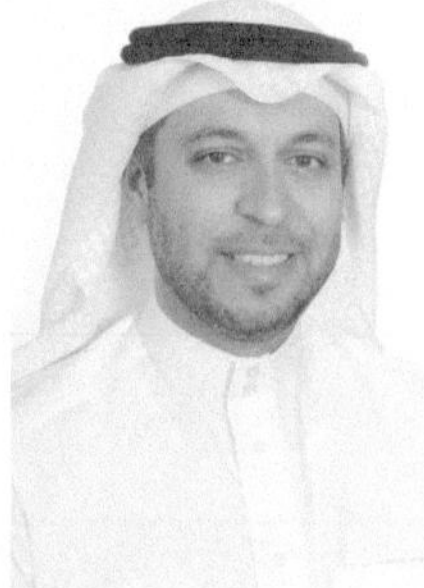

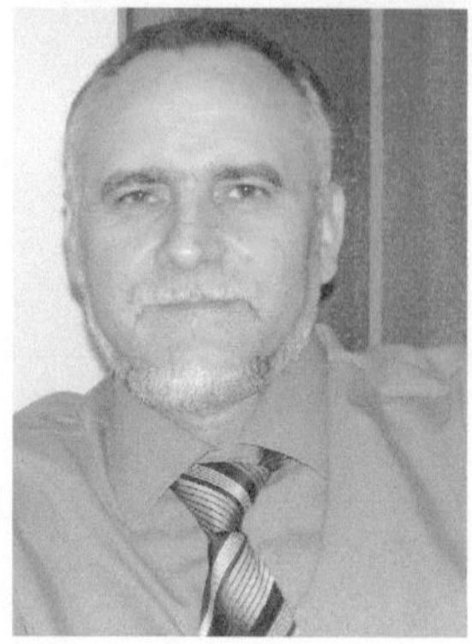

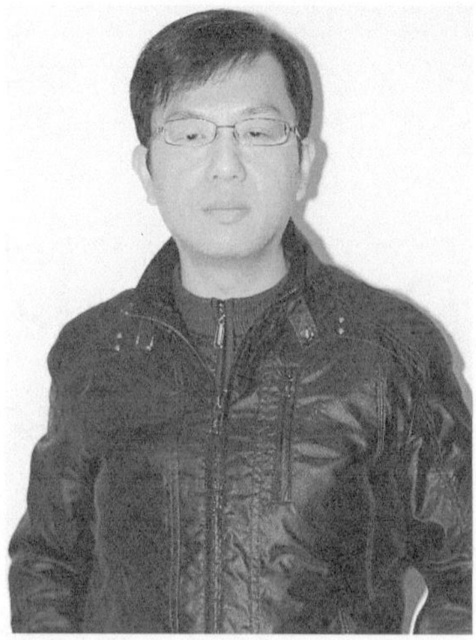

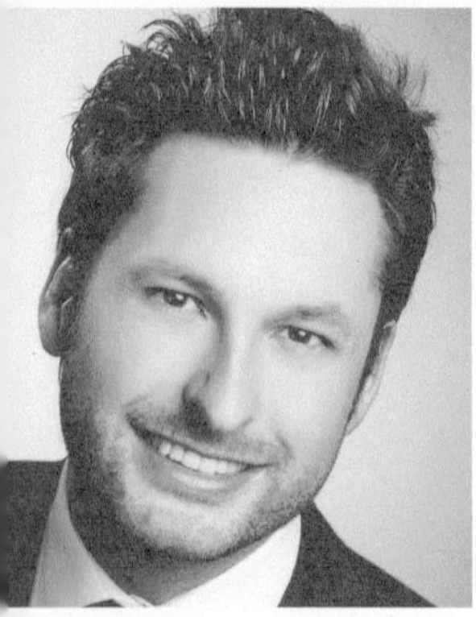

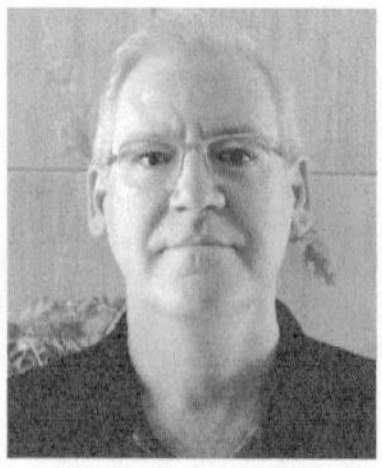

IntechOpen

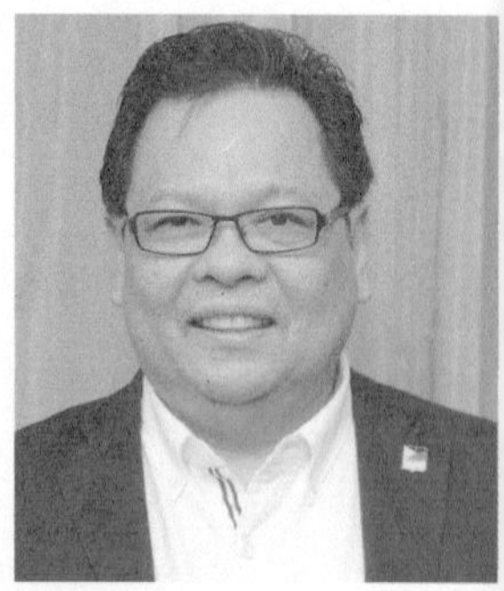

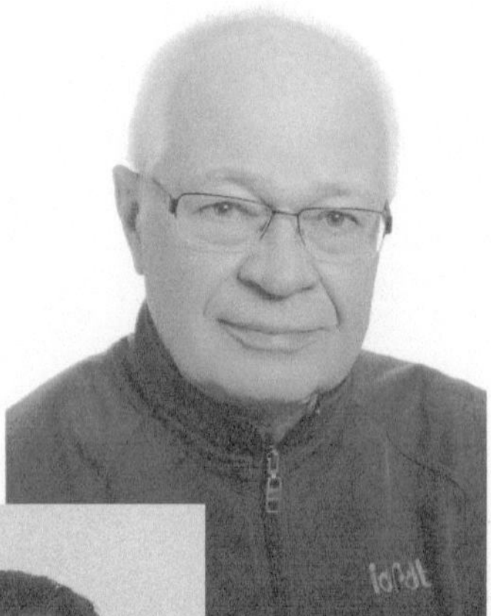

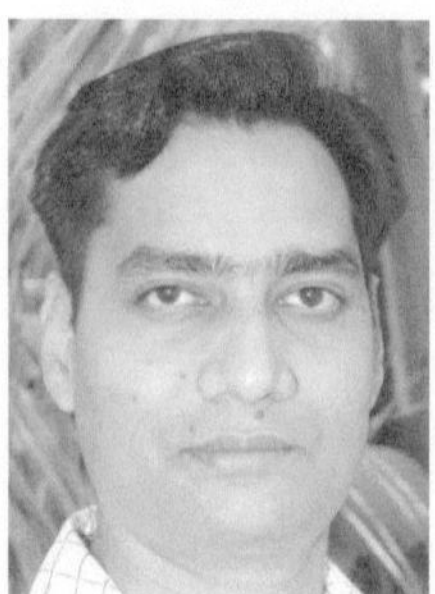

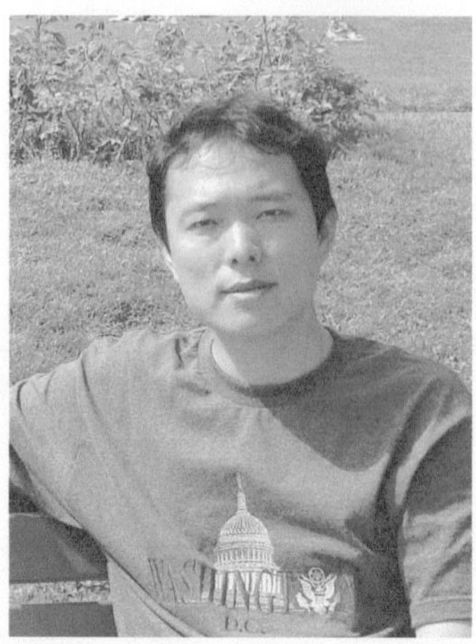

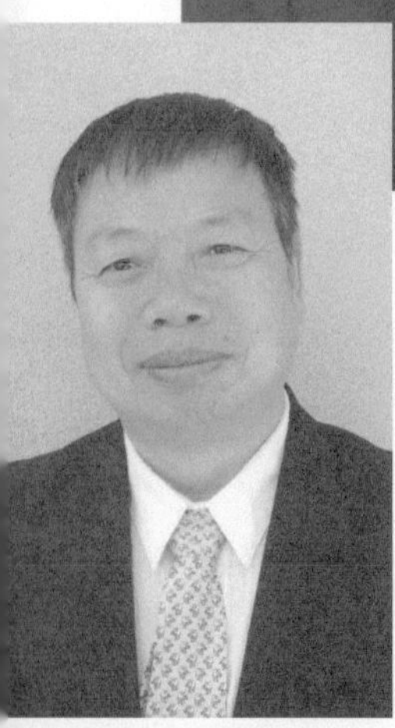

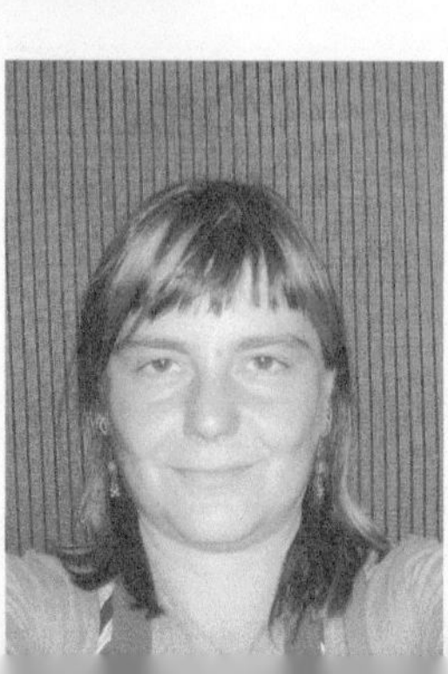

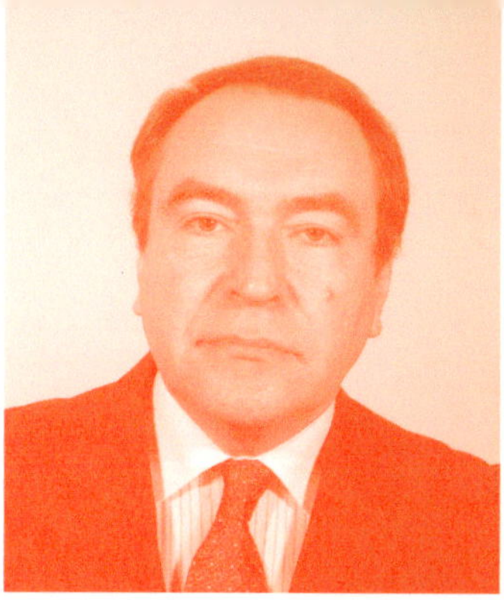
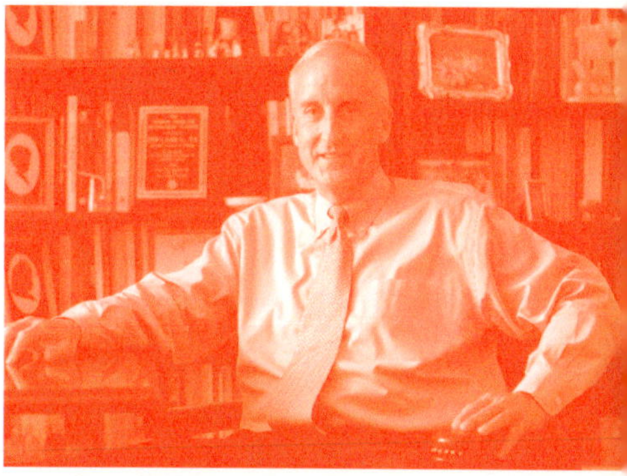
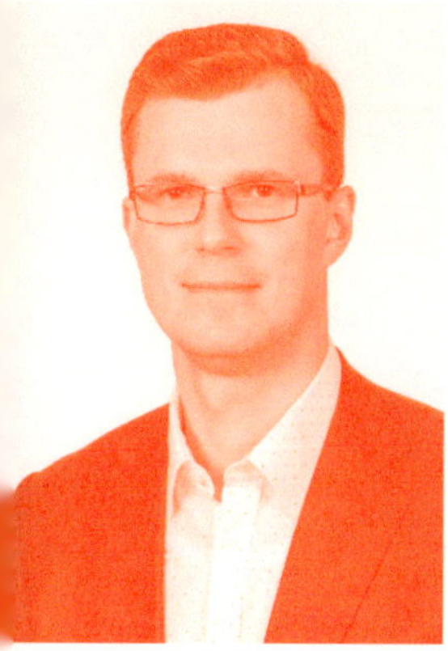
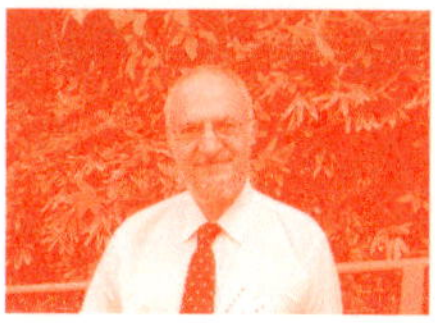
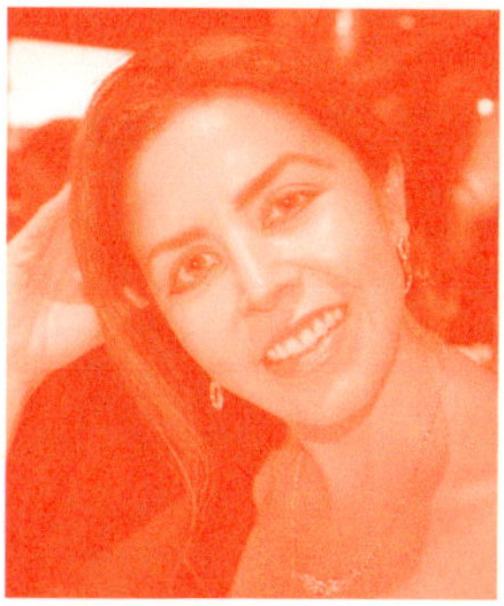

Supporting open minds since 2005

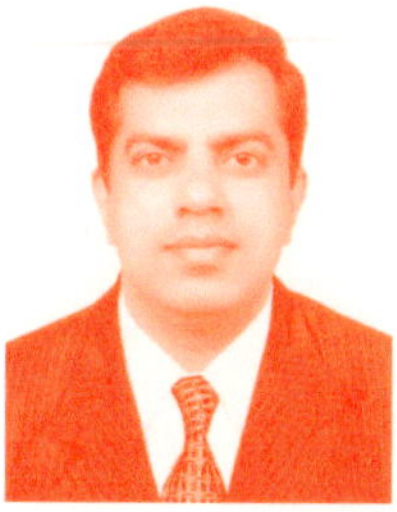
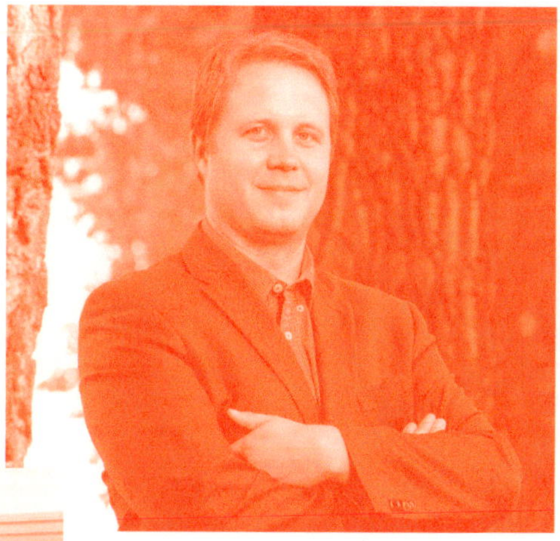
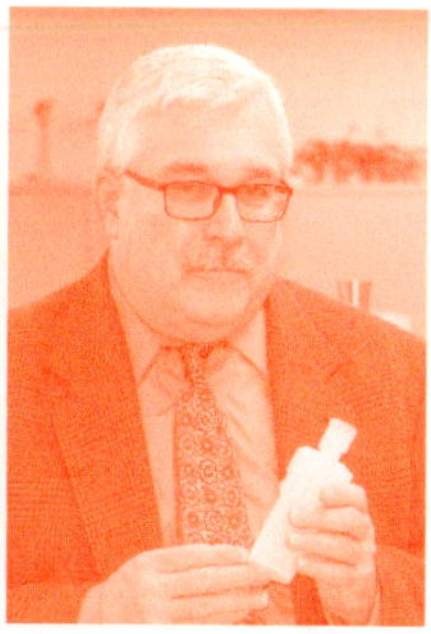
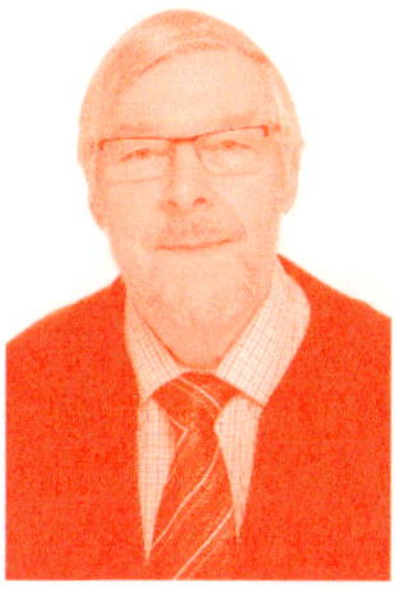
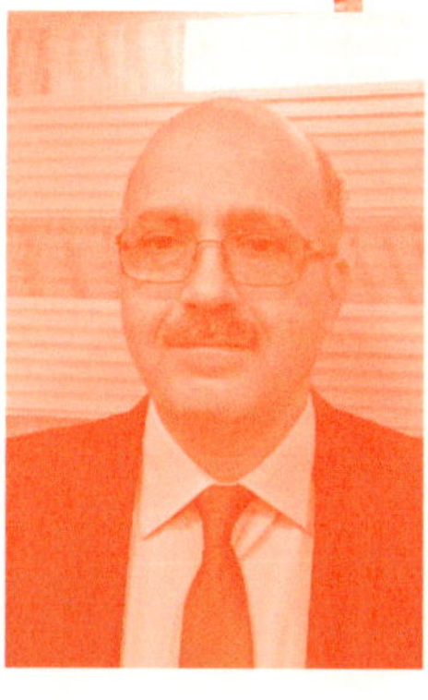
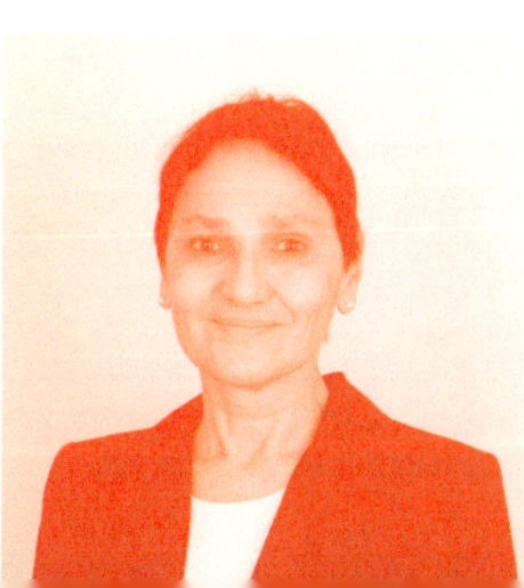
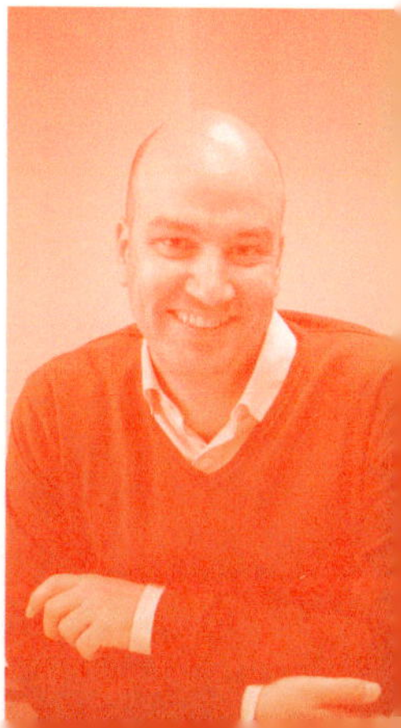

Diverticular Disease of the Colon - Recent Knowledge of Physiopathology, Endoscopic Approaches, Clinical and Surgical Treatments
http://dx.doi.org/10.5772/intechopen.94689
Edited by José Joaquim Ribeiro da Rocha and Marley Ribeiro Feitosa

Contributors
Cristian Mesina, Theodor Viorel Dumitrescu, Cosmin Vasile Obleaga, Mihai Calin Ciorbagiu, Mihaela-Iustina Mesina Botoran, Rafael Luporini, Marcel Domeniconi, Ana Carolina Parra, André Rizzo, Daniela Freitas, Sthefânia Frizol, Antonio Tursi, Mariana Morales-Cruz, Paulina Moctezuma Velázquez, Jeremy Meyer, Frédéric Ris, Luciano Dias de Oliveira Reis, Marcos Ricardo da Silva Rodrigues, Celso Augusto Milani Cardoso Filho, Cassiana Franco Dias dos Reis, Alex Antonio de Paula Costa, José Joaquim Joaquim Ribeiro Da Rocha, Marley Feitosa

First published in London, United Kingdom, 2022 by IntechOpen
IntechOpen is the global imprint of INTECHOPEN LIMITED, registered in England and Wales, registration number: 11086078, 5 Princes Gate Court, London, SW7 2QJ, United Kingdom
Printed in Croatia

British Library Cataloguing-in-Publication Data
A catalogue record for this book is available from the British Library

Additional hard and PDF copies can be obtained from orders@intechopen.com

Diverticular Disease of the Colon - Recent Knowledge of Physiopathology, Endoscopic Approaches, Clinical and Surgical Treatments
Edited by José Joaquim Ribeiro da Rocha and Marley Ribeiro Feitosa
p. cm.
Print ISBN 978-1-83968-578-1
Online ISBN 978-1-83968-579-8
eBook (PDF) ISBN 978-1-83968-580-4

For EU product safety concerns:
IN TECH d.o.o., Prolaz Marije Krucifikse Kozulić 3, 51000 Rijeka, Croatia, info@intechopen.com or visit our website at intechopen.com.

Meet the editors

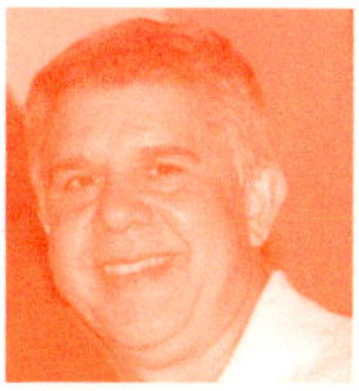

Dr. José Joaquim Ribeiro da Rocha is a Professor of Surgery, Faculty of Medicine, University of São Paulo, Brazil. He is also the director of the Division of Coloproctology of the Department of Surgery and Anatomy of the Faculty of Medicine of Ribeirão Preto, University of São Paulo. Dr. da Rocha has conducted research on diffuse peritonitis, intestinal anastomosis, and transanal endoscopic operations. He is the editor of *Coloproctology - Principles and Practices*, which is now in its second edition. He earned a master's degree and Ph.D. in Surgery at the Department of Surgery and Anatomy, University of São Paulo. He is also a coloproctology surgeon at Hospital São Paulo.

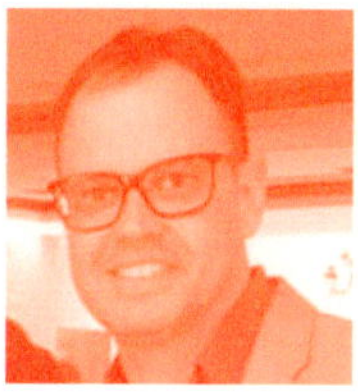

Dr. Marley Ribeiro Feitosa is a surgeon at the Ribeirão Preto Medical School, University of São Paulo, Brazil, where he earned a Ph.D. in Surgery. He currently carries out teaching and research activities at the same university. He is also in private practice at Proctogastroclínica, São Paulo, Brazil.

Contents

Preface

This book reviews and updates information on the diverticular disease of the colon. It covers all relevant aspects of the disease, including anatomy, etiopathogenesis, symptoms, diagnosis, colonoscopy, complications, and treatment.

The introductory chapter presents the historical evolution, anatomy, and etiopathogenesis of colonic diverticular disease. It also discusses clinical diagnosis, differential diagnosis, and pertinent imaging tests. It highlights the main inflammatory and hemorrhagic complications, their stages, and therapeutic aspects.

Chapter 2 presents concepts, etiopathogenesis, and clinical and epidemiological conditions of segmental colitis associated with diverticular disease, as well as discusses clinical, laboratory, and radiological diagnosis of this condition. It also proposes a classification of segmental colitis and an algorithm for treatment and clinical follow-up.

Chapters 3 and 4 discuss the complicated diverticular disease, classified according to the severity and taking into account tomographic aspects and surgical findings. These chapters also examine therapeutic approaches and provide extensive photographic documentation.

Chapter 5 provides an update on antibiotic therapy in acute diverticulitis. It includes an extensive literary survey with relevant conclusions about when antibiotic therapy should be indicated in acute diverticulitis.

Finally, Chapter 6 discusses colonoscopic investigation after acute diverticulitis and presents interesting conclusions about the need to endoscopically evaluate the colon after diagnosis.

I decided to edit this book because of my direct relationship with diverticular disease of the colon throughout my professional life, both in the Faculty of Medicine next to the public hospital where hundreds of patients are assisted and/or operated on, as well as in the private sector where I've practiced as a coloproctologist for more than thirty years.

I'd like to thank my co-editor, Dr. Marley F. Ribeiro, who is also a practicing surgeon as well as a teacher and lecturer. I am also grateful to IntechOpen for the opportunity to participate in this book project. This volume will guide many people in the diagnostic and therapeutic management of the diverticular disease.

José Joaquim Ribeiro da Rocha
Associate Professor of Department of Anatomy and Surgery,
Faculty of Medicine of Ribeirão Preto,
University of Sao Paulo,
Brazil

Marley Ribeiro Feitosa, MD, PhD
Division of Coloproctology,
Departament of Surgery and Anatomy,
Ribeirão Preto Medical School,
University of São Paulo,
Brazil

Section 1

Introduction

Chapter 1

Introductory Chapter: Diverticule Disease of the Colon—DDC

José Joaquim Ribeiro da Rocha and Marley Ribeiro Feitosa

1. Introduction

This book is intended to review, update and bring a wide knowledge of the diverticular disease of the colon and its own relationships in search of better driving in diagnosis and treating this morbity so frequently in our media.

In this chapter introducing the book, we have an approach of all the relevant aspects with respect to anatomy, etiopathogenesis, symptoms, diagnosis, complications and treatment of diverticular colon disease. In the following chapters, the other authors present their experiences and their research on specific topics related to diverticular colon disease.

2. General considerations about colon diverticular disease

The large intestine diverticules are small hernias on the wall of the large intestine, composed of mucosa and submucosa that inherit by the lay of the smooth intestine musculature (**Figures 1–3**).

Colonic diverticulum is acquired, and pulsional diverticula are under the influence of increased intraluminal pressure, which promotes mucous herniations that

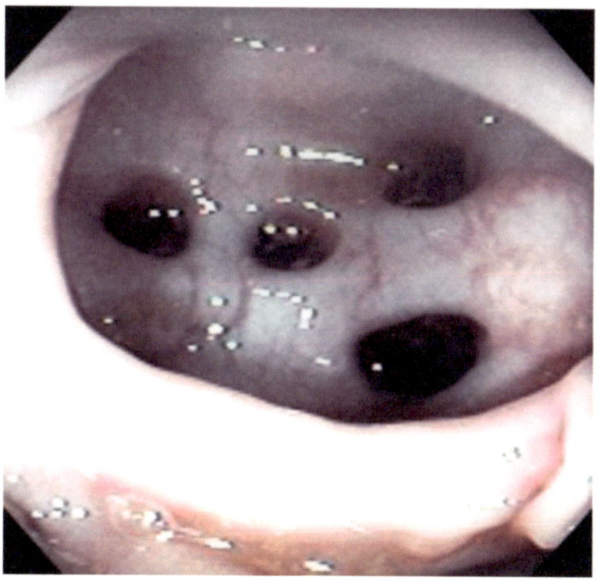

Figure 1.
Diverticules—internal vision by the colic lumen.

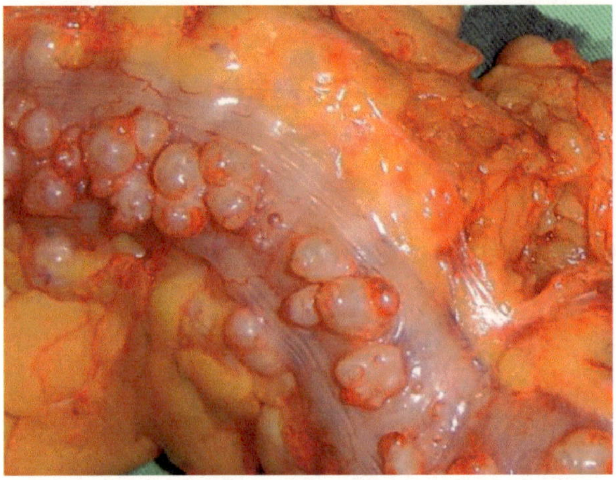

Figure 2.
Diverticules—external vision by the serosa surface of the colon.

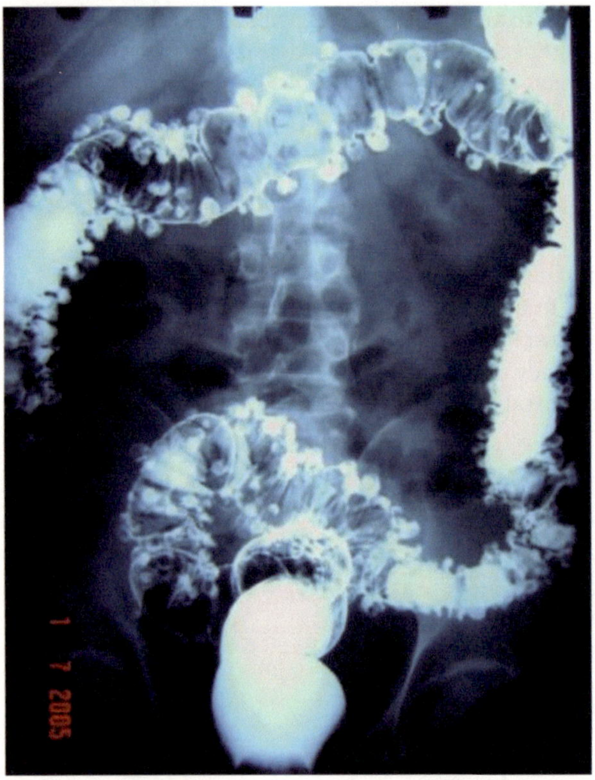

Figure 3.
Pancolonic diverticular disease.

protrude through points of weakness in the intestinal wall where blood vessels enter (**Figures 4** and **5**).

Several authors, since 1849, have been pioneers in the description of the diverticules on the intestine wall, among them are Cruveilhier, Haberson and Sidney Jones [1–4].

The history of diverticular disease can be divided into some phases according to Painter and Burkitt [5].

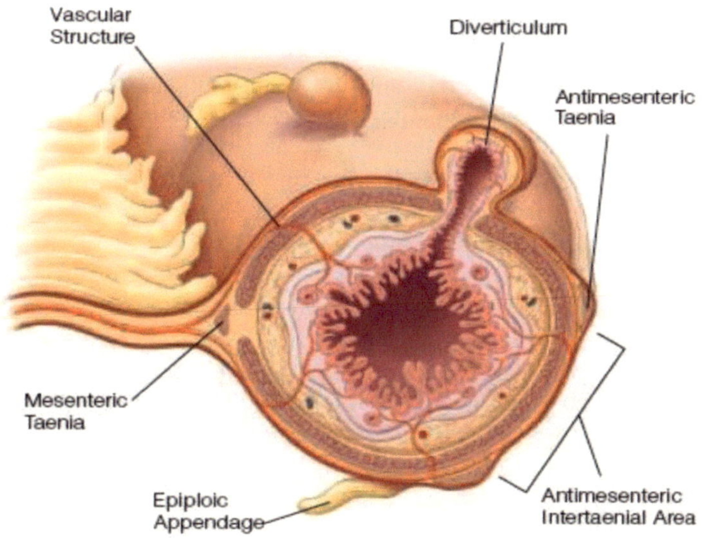

Figure 4.
Anatomy of a colonic diverticulum.

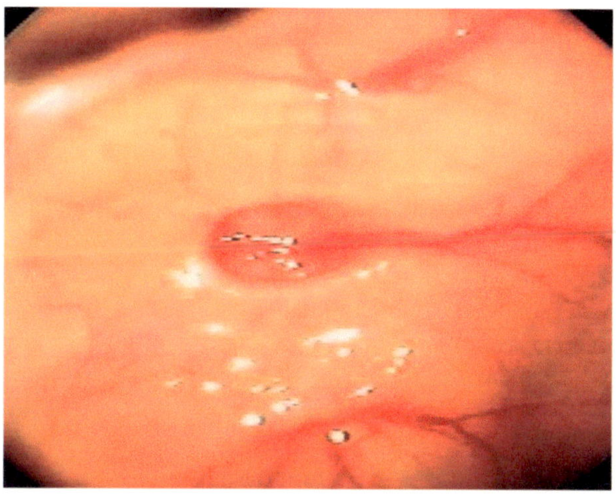

Figure 5.
Penetrating vessel in the diverticular ostium.

- Illness as a curiosity
- Recognition of the disease as a clinical problem
- Diverticular disease as a growing problem
- Surgical intervention for its treatment
- Etiopathogenesis involving the muscles of the intestinal wall

Consider a Western man's disease, 30% of cases affect people up to 60 years old and 60% up to 80 years old. From the fifth to the ninth decade of life, the incidence ranges from 5 to 50% of the general population.

The great majority of patients are asymptomatic (75%), in young people, under 50 years, the evolution is usually more aggressive and in the elderly over 60 years, there is a greater risk of hemorrhage. Urgent surgery occurs in about 5% of cases [6, 7]. Over time, new knowledge about etiopathogenics, its complications, diagnosis and treatment was discovered [8–10].

There is no specific cause. Physiopathology is based on the hypertonia of the smooth musculature of the intestinal wall with increased intraluminal pressure of the large intestine, favoring this hernia on the intestine wall.

Since the twentieth century, the incidence of DDC, whether by the clinical and laboratory diagnosis or by the finding of autopsies, is more common in industrialized countries and less frequent in developing countries [11].

As a degenerative disease is considered in the intestine wall, it is most frequent over 50 years of age, but there are cases in younger individuals. There is no significant relationship as to gender, but there is as to family background, that is, hereditarity.

The etiopathogenesis of DDC has been related to factors such as the poor fiber diet, changes in colon motility, collagen function in the intestine wall, genetics and age [12, 13].

In recent reviews, it has been speculated about the enteric nervous system in DDC [14].

Inflammation is the most common manifestation (diverticulitis), which is much more frequent in the diverticulum of the sigmoid colon. Diverticulitis can be acute, the most common form; however, there are patients who present the chronic form, with periods of acute inflammation.

In the natural history of acute diverticulitis, symptoms affect approximately 10 to 25% of patients with diverticular disease. The sigmoid is involved in 90% of cases. There is a palpable mass in 20% of cases. The incidence increases with age and mostly responds to treatment with clinical measures.

Seizures are recurrent 30 to 60% of the time, 50% in the first year and 90% up to 5 years later.

About 70 to 80% have intermittent symptoms, and about 25% after the first hospitalization will require a new hospitalization.

There is surgical indication in 10 to 30% of cases. Complicated forms appear 25% of the time after the first attack and 60% of the time after the second attack [15, 16].

Diagnosis is based on physical and image examinations and colonoscopy, opportunely indicated.

Computerized tomography is the examination of choice for uncomplicated acute diverticulitis and also complicated diverticulitis with high sensitivity and specificity (**Figure 6**). Colonoscopy must be avoided in the acute inflammatory activity phase due to perforation risk but must be carried out after the acute framework resolution to exclude other injuries such as colorectal neoplasms [17, 18].

Acute diverticulitis complicated with surgical indication depending on the stage well established by Hinchey [19] (**Figures** 7 and **8**).

The patient's systemic state will direct it to make a stoma or not [20–22].

In the differential diagnosis of acute diverticulitis, there are several pathologies such as: acute appendicitis, Crohn's disease, gastroenterocolitis, colorectalcancer, intestinal obstruction of another origin, ischemic colitis, gynecological disorders, Meckel's diverticulitis appendagites, lithiasis and/or urinary infection and irritable bowel syndrome [23, 24].

Other less frequent ways of presentation are complicated acute and/or chronic diverticulitis, with abdominal abscess (**Figures 9** and **10**), peritonitis, perforation (**Figure 11**), bladder, vagine and cutaneous fistulas (**Figures 12** and **13**). Another complication is stenosis (**Figure 14**), caused by fibrosis and inducing intestinal obstruction [7, 25].

DOI: http://dx.doi.org/10.5772/intechopen.101573

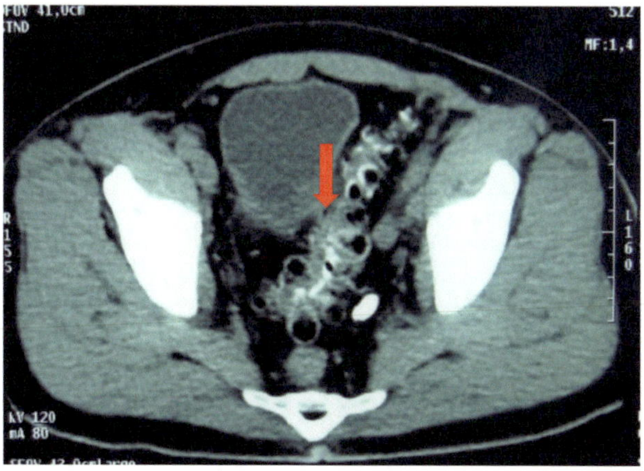

Figure 6.
Acute diverticulitis with thickening of the wall, blurring of pericolic fat and adherence to the bladder wall.

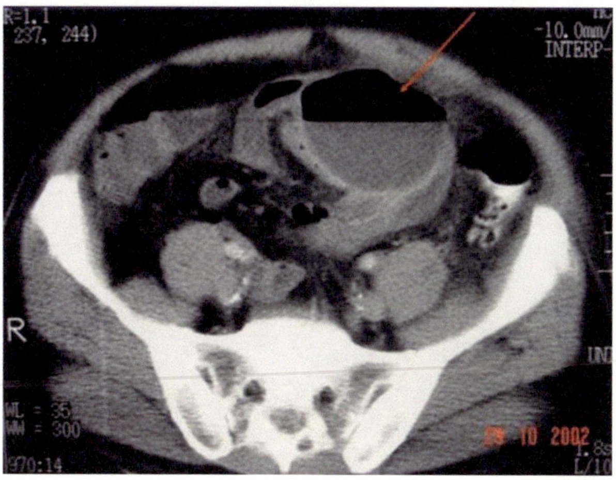

Figure 7.
Hinchey II—large abdominal abscess.

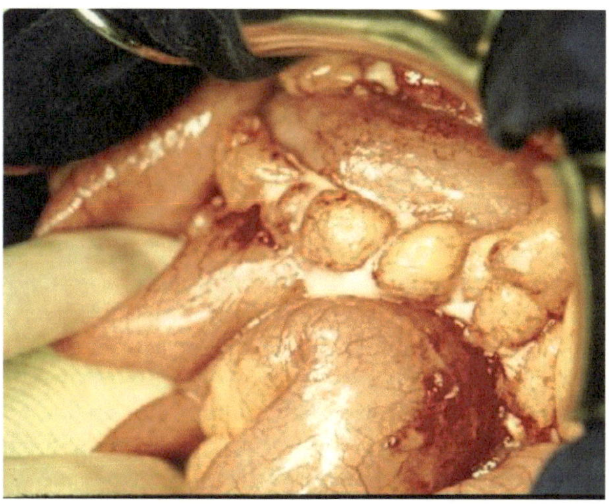

Figure 8.
Hinchey III—diverticulitis with purulent peritonitis.

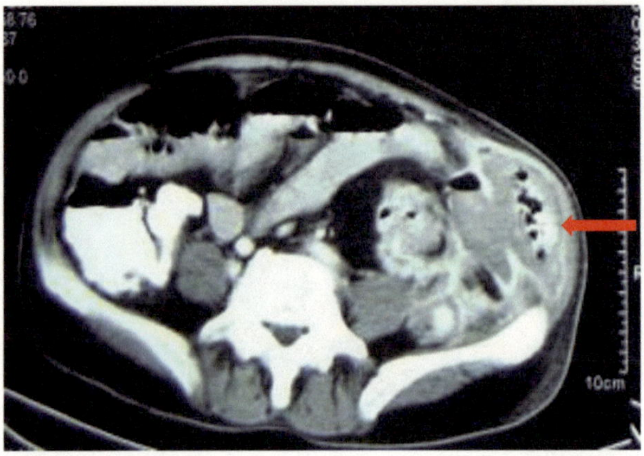

Figure 9.
Diverticular diseases abscess pericolic—left flank.

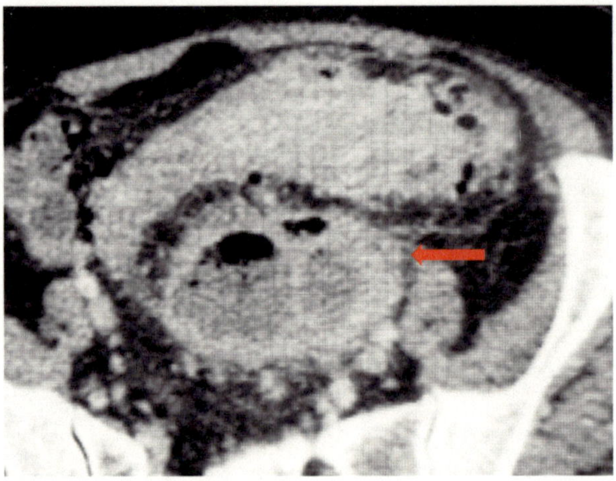

Figure 10.
Diverticular diseases abscess pericolic—left iliac fossa.

From the anatomic and clinical point of view, we can divide diverticular disease in hypertonic diverticular disease, restricted to the sigmoid colon where the biggest complications occur, habitually accomplishing the youngest individuals until seventh decade. The other way, hypothonic called is when all the large intestine is involved and in this case, the main complication is the enterorragia, accommodating elderly individuals. There are patients who present the two forms [26, 27].

The most frequent cause of lower gastrointestinal bleeding in patients over 60 years of age is colonic diverticular disease. It occurs most frequently in the right colon where the ostia and cupola of the diverticula are wider and thinner and therefore have greater exposure of the penetrating vessels. About 50 to 90% bleed in the right and transverse colon. About 20% of patients with diverticular disease may bleed over their lifetime. About 25% may have recurrent bleeding and 5% may have massive bleeding. About 80% of the time the bleeding stops spontaneously.

Of those patients who need more than four units of blood a day, 60% will need urgent surgery. During rare blood-type situations, transfusion difficulties, rebleeding after bleeding has stopped, and massive transfusions and when blood loss is greater than replacement, colectomy is indicated. The postoperative mortality rate is 9%.

Surgery depends on the location of the bleeding point, which can be investigated by scintigraphy, arteriography or colonoscopy (**Figure 15**).

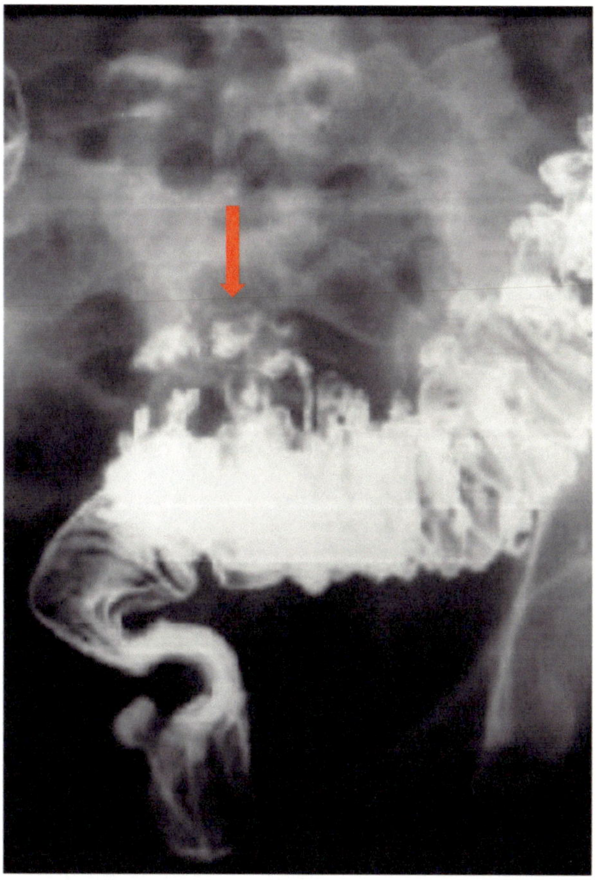

Figure 11.
Diverticular disease perfuration.

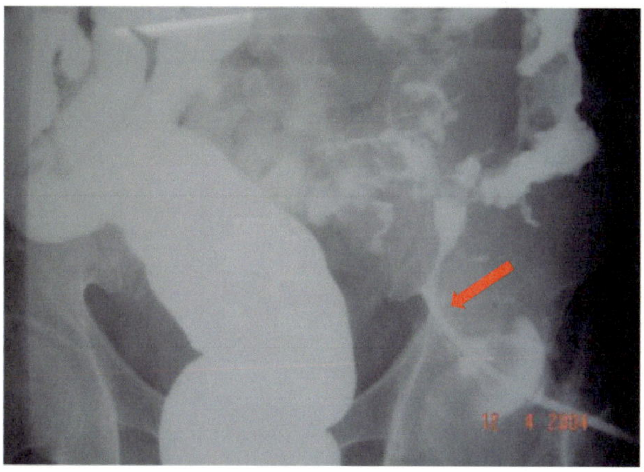

Figure 12.
Perfuration and fistula colo-cutaneous.

Three conditions are important in deciding which surgery to perform: 1. Clinical conditions and patient characteristics. 2. Experience of the surgeon. 3. Location of bleeding.

The ideal surgery is segmental or total colectomy with an ileum colon or an ileum rectus anastomosis.

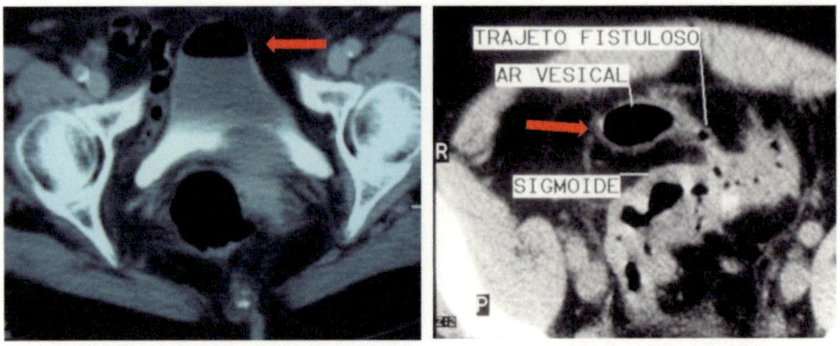

Figure 13.
Sigmoid—vesical fistula air in the top of the bladder.

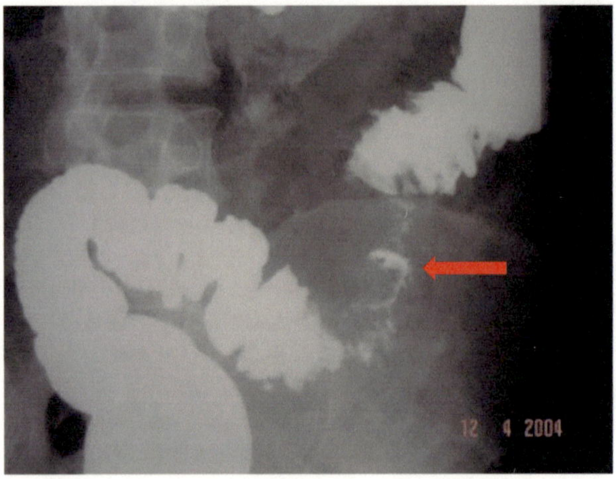

Figure 14.
Diverticular diseases stenosis of the sigmoid colon.

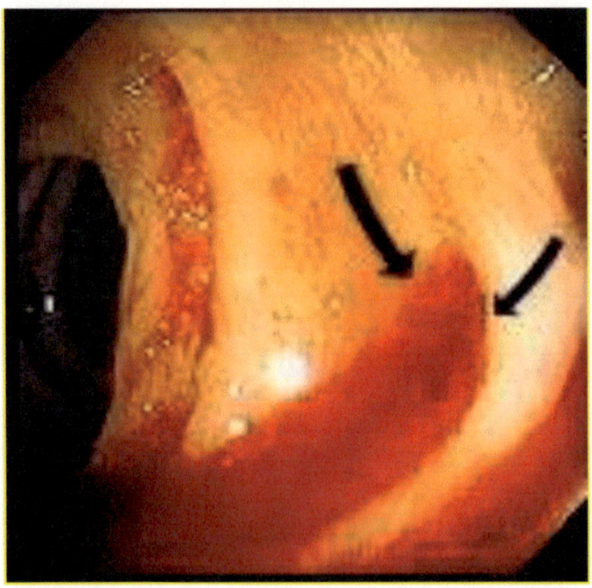

Figure 15.
Colonoscopy showing the point of bleeding from diverticulum.

The likely surgery is total colectomy with ileum rectus anastomosis and protective ileostomy. The safest surgery is total colectomy with terminal ileostomy and burial of the rectal stump (**Figure 16**) [28–30].

An atypical presentation is segmental colitis associated with diverticular disease (SCAD), inflammatory disease that mimics inflammatory bowel diseases with variable intensity from slight to deep ulcerations (**Figure 17**) and which requires adequate cure treatment [31–33].

Prevention of complications, food and personal habits are controversial topics and this book hopes to help in this clarification.

Clinical or surgical treatment is guided by symptoms and complications [34–38].

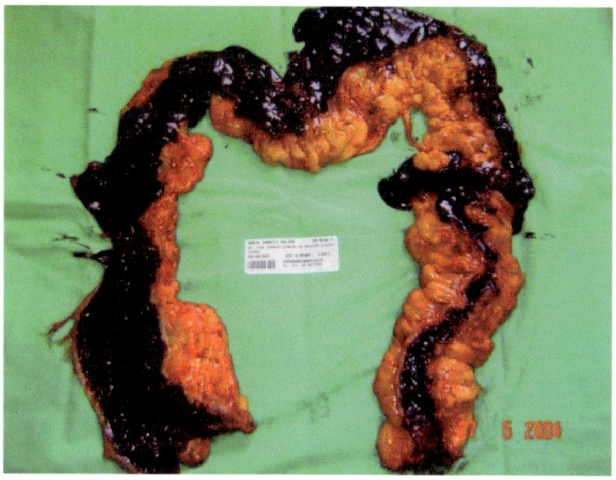

Figure 16.
Diverticular diseases pancolectomy for severe hemorrhage.

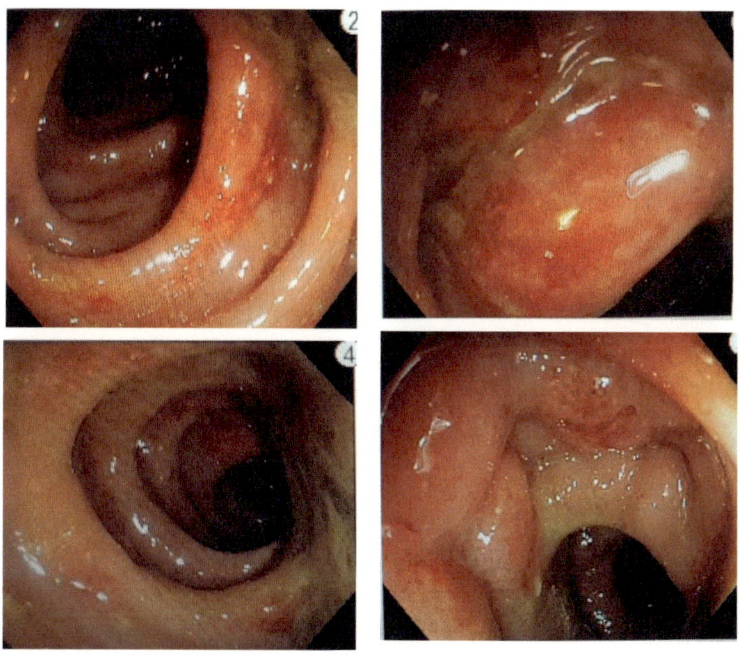

Figure 17.
Sigmoid segmental colitis (edema + hiperemia + ulcerations).

Author details

José Joaquim Ribeiro da Rocha[1*] and Marley Ribeiro Feitosa[2]

1 USP Medical School, Ribeirao Preto, Brazil

2 Faculty of Medicine of USP, Ribeirao Preto, Brazil

*Address all correspondence to: ribeiro.rocha0717@gmail.com

References

[1] Cruveilhier J. Traitê d'Anatomic Pathologique. Paris, Balliére. 1849;**1**:593

[2] Goligher J, editor. Surgery of the Anus, Rectum and Colon. 5th ed. London: Ballière Tindall; 1985. p. 1083

[3] Hansemann, Nauwerck e Graser. Arch Klin Chir. 1892;**59**:638

[4] Kirschner M, Nordmann O. Cirurgia del Abdomen. 2ª ed. Barcelona: Editoria Labor; 1946. p. 751

[5] Painter NS, Burkitt DP. Diverticular disease of the colon: A deficiency disease of Western civilization. British Medical Journal. 1971;**2**:450-454

[6] Schoetz D. Diverticular disease of the colon: A century-old problem. Diseases of the Colon and Rectum. 1999;**42**:703-709

[7] Parks TG. Natural history of diverticular disease of the colon. Clinics in Gastroenterology. 1975;**4**:53-69

[8] World Gastroenterology Organisation (WGO). Practice Guidelines. Geneva: Diverticular Disease; 2007.

[9] Garibay RR et al. Guias clínicas de diagnostico y tratamento de la enfermedad diverticular del colon. Etiologia, fisiopatologia, epidemilogía: em México y el mundo. Revista de Gastroenterología de México. 2008;**73**(4):255-257

[10] Vermeulen J et al. Pathophysiology and prevention of diverticulitis and perforation. Netherlands Journal of Medicine. 2010;**68**(10):303-309

[11] Segal L, Leibowitz B. The distributional pattern of diverticular disease. Diseases of the Colon and Rectum. 1989;**32**:227-229

[12] Commane D et al. Diet, ageing and genetic factors in the pathogenesis of diverticular disease. World Journal of Gastroenterology. 2009;**25**(20): 2479-2488

[13] Bassotti G, Chistolini F, Morelli A. Pathophysiological aspecto f diverticular disease of colon and role of large bowel motility. World Journal of Gastroenterology. 2003;**9**:2140-2149

[14] Knowles CH et al. New perspectives in the diagnosis and management of enteric neuropathies. Nature Reviews. Gastroenterology & Hepatology. 2013;**10**(4):206-218

[15] Bogardus ST Jr. What do we know about diverticular disease? A brief overview. Journal of Clinical Gastroenterology. 2006;**40**:108-111

[16] Rafferty J, Shellito P, Hyman NH, et al. Practice parameters for sigmoid diverticulitis. Diseases of the Colon and Rectum. 2006;**49**:939-944

[17] Ambrosetti P. Value of CT for acute diverticulitis. Digestive Diseases. 2012;**30**:51-55

[18] Bar-Meir S, Lahat A, Melzer E. Role of endoscopy in patients with diverticualr disease. Digestive Diseases. 2012;**30**: 60-63

[19] Hinchey EJ, Schjall PG, Richards GK. Treatment of perforated diverticular disease of the colon. Advances Surgery. 1978;**12**(12):85-109

[20] Janes SE, Meagher A, Frizelle FA. Management of diverticulitis. BMJ. 2006;**332**(7536):271-275

[21] Colecchia A et al. Diverticular disease of the colon: New perspective in symptom development and treatment. World Journal of Gastroenterology. 2003;**7**:1385-1389

[22] Roxburg RA, Dawson JL, Yeo L. Emergency resection in treatment of

diverticular disease of colon complicated by peritonitis. British Journal of Medicine. 1968;**3**(5616):465-466

[23] World Gastroenteroloy Organisagion (WGO). Practice Guidelines. Diverticular Disease. 2007.

[24] Garibay RR et al. Guias clinicas de diagnostico y tratamento de la enfermedad diverticular del colon. Etiologia, fisiopatologia, emidemiología: em México y el mundo. Revista de Gastroenterología de México 2008; 73($): 255-257.

[25] Nader FBI, Hellwig B, Nader LA. Doença diverticular. In: Moraes-Filho JPP, editor. Tratado das enfermidades gastrointestinais e pancreática. 1st ed. São Paulo: Roca; 2008. pp. 982-989

[26] Floch MH, White JÁ. Management of diverticular disease is changing. World Journal of Gastroenterology. 2006;**12**(20):3225-3228

[27] Salzman H, Lilie D. Diverticular disease: Diagnosis and treatment. American Family Physician. 2005;**72**(7): 1229-1234

[28] Wilkins T et al. Diverticular bleeding. American Family Physician. 2009;**80**(9):977-983

[29] Barnet J, Messmann H. Diagnosis and management of lower gastrointestinal bleeding. Nature Reviews Gastro-enterology & Hepatology. 2009;**6**: 637-646

[30] Poncet G et al. Natural history of acute colonic diverticular bleeding: a prospective study in 133 consecutive patients. Alimentary Pharmacology & Therapeutics. 2010;**32**:466-471

[31] Koutroubakis IE, Antoniou P, Tzardi M, Kouroumalis EA. International Journal of Colorectal Disease. 2005;**20**: 28-32

[32] Harpaz N, Sachar DB. Segmental colitis associated with diverticular disease and other IDG look-alikes. Journal of Clinical Gastroenterology. 2006;**40**:132-135

[33] Tursi A, Elisei W, Brandimarte G. The endoscopic spectrum of segmental colitis associated wth diverticulosis. Colorectal Disease. 1010;**12**:464-470

[34] Golder M et al. Demographic determinants of risk, colon distribution and density scores of diverticualr disease. World Journal of Gastroenterology. 2011;**17**:109-117

[35] Etzioni DA et al. Diverticulitis in the Unites States 1998-2005: changing patterns of disease and treatment. Annals of Surgery. 2009;**249**:210-217

[36] Painter NS, Burkitt DP. Diverticular disease of the colon, a 20th century problem. Clinics in Gastroenterology. 1975;**4**:3-21

[37] Aldoori WH et al. A prospective study of diet and the risk of symptomatic diverticular disease in men. The American Journal of Clinical Nutrition. 1994;**60**:757-764

[38] Bafutto M, Oliveira EC. Doença Diverticular dos Cólons. 3ª.ed. ed. Brazil: Office Editora e Publicidade Ltda; 2016. p. 481

Section 2

Colitis and Diverticular Diseases of the Colon

Chapter 2

Segmental Colitis Associated with Diverticulosis

Rafael Luís Luporini, Marcel Domeniconi,
Ana Carolina Parra, André Rizzo, Daniela Freitas,
Sthefânia Frizol and Antonio Tursi

Abstract

Segmental colitis associated with diverticulosis is a pathology of recent knowledge, whose pathogenesis is still poorly defined. Diagnosis is mainly based on colonoscopy and histopathological study. Clinical features are chronic diarrhea, abdominal cramps in the lower right quadrant, and intermittent hematochezia. The diagnosis is evidenced by colonoscopy showing inflammation in the colic mucosa between the diverticula, sparing the diverticular orifice associated with an anatomopathological condition showing chronic inflammation. The involvement is preferably sigmoid and may involve a descending colon, sparing the rectum. The treatment is similar to that of inflammatory bowel diseases in mild forms, but recent studies have presented new alternatives with good results. The treatment is not yet well defined, and antibiotics, mesalamine, and corticoid therapy can be used, and surgery can even be performed for refractory cases.

Keywords: segmental colitis associated with diverticulosis, diverticular disease, inflammatory bowel diseases

1. Introduction

Colonic diverticular disease occurs in over 60% of people over 60 in the West. It can present various forms of manifestation, from asymptomatic conditions detected in endoscopic or imaging exams, to cases of acute diverticulitis, with a pericolic inflammatory process originating in a diverticulum and spreading to adjacent tissues due to micro-perforations [1, 2].

Segmental colitis associated with diverticulosis (SCAD) is a chronic inflammatory change that occurs in colonic mucosal segments between colonic diverticula, limited to the sigmoid and left colon, generally not affecting the diverticular ostium [2–6]. Rectum and right colon are spared from any endoscopic and histological inflammation [5, 6]. It is a recently recognized pathology within the spectrum of manifestations of colonic diverticular disease [7].

The inflammation of the colonic mucosa may resemble other inflammatory bowel diseases (IBD) [Crohn's disease (CD) and ulcerative colitis (UC)] in both clinical and endoscopic aspects [3, 7, 8]. Inflammation is non-specific, non-granulomatous, and localized. It appears to be a self-limited inflammatory process [3, 9].

2. Terminology

Several terms have been used to refer to this pathology, including crescentic fold disease, colitis associated with diverticular disease, diverticular colitis, diverticular-associated colitis (DAC), or segmental colitis associated with diverticulosis (SCAD), this being the most currently accepted [3, 9].

3. Pathogenesis

The exact pathogenic mechanism is not known, but it appears to be multifactorial pathogenesis [10]. Several hypotheses have been raised, including mucosal prolapse leading to mucosal ischemia, fecal stasis within diverticula, and consequent dysbiosis that can trigger an immune response, and high exposure to intraluminal antigens and toxins [3–5, 11].

4. Epidemiology

It is a rare pathology, with a prevalence ranging from 0.3 to 1.3% of patients undergoing colonoscopy [7] and 1.15 to 11.4% of patients with colonic diverticula.

The mean age at diagnosis is 61.7 to 66.5 years, similar to the mean age of onset of diverticular disease of the colon [3, 4]. There is also a predominance of males (58.7%) [4, 9].

5. Associated factors

SCAD is believed to be associated with several factors, including changes in intestinal motility, bacterial stasis in the colon, bacterial overgrowth, and inflammation [3].

6. Clinical condition

Although SCAD is still considered a pathology among the spectrum of diverticular diseases, it differs from diverticulitis (which is the inflammation of a diverticulum). As consequence, also the clinical picture is different.

The clinical picture associated with SCAD is variable, with studies citing complaints of diarrhea, rectal bleeding (live or with other changes), abdominal pain, and tenesmus [3, 4, 10]. Fever and weight loss are rare [4]. More than a third of patients have at least two associated symptoms at diagnosis [12].

The clinical picture can be very similar to that of mild inflammatory bowel disease. Occasionally, the patient may be asymptomatic, and the diagnosis is made only at random during colonoscopy for another reason.

Symptoms may vary according to the subtype of SCAD presented, with diarrhea being more common in type A and rectal bleeding in types C and D [12]. Type B presents with more than one symptom 39% of the time, with diarrhea and rectal bleeding being the main ones. Abdominal pain is more frequent in types C and D [2].

7. Laboratory and radiological exams

Laboratory tests (blood count, white blood count, erythrocyte sedimentation rate, C-reactive protein, fecal inflammatory markers, fecal calprotectin) and radiological tests do not show specific results, but help to exclude differential diagnoses [4, 13].

Computed tomography may show thickening of the colonic wall in a colon segment with pre-existing diverticulosis. Fat blurring can be seen occasionally [14].

8. Diagnosis

The diagnosis of SCAD must initially be performed excluding other pathologies that cause intestinal inflammation, among these differential diagnoses: ischemic colitis, colitis induced by anti-inflammatory drugs, infectious colitis (mainly cytomegalovirus and Clostridium difficile), and IBD [3]. SCAD can mimic clinical and endoscopic presentations of IBD [10], and some pictures are indistinguishable from IBD [7].

Colonoscopy is the mainstay for the diagnosis of SCAD [15]. By its use, inflammation restricted to the mucosa between the diverticula is detected, sparing the diverticular orifice [3, 4]. Inflammation basically affects the sigmoid colon and left colon with normal mucosa in the rest of the colon (**Figure 1**).

It is indicated to perform biopsies of affected areas and normal areas to accurately locate inflammatory changes [15]. It is also suggested to perform a rectal biopsy (whose result should be negative) to strengthen the diagnosis [3, 7]. The pathologist must be informed about the clinical suspicion for better elucidation of the case.

Histopathologically, SCAD presents an active inflammatory infiltrate, similar to ulcerative colitis, unlike colonic diverticular disease, which presents a nonspecific inflammatory infiltrate, sometimes active, but different from those of inflammatory bowel diseases [5, 16, 17].

Therefore, it is concluded that the diagnosis must include colonoscopy and histopathological examination, confirming the inflammatory process in the affected area, and ruling out inflammation in other areas, in addition to laboratory and imaging tests excluding other pathologies.

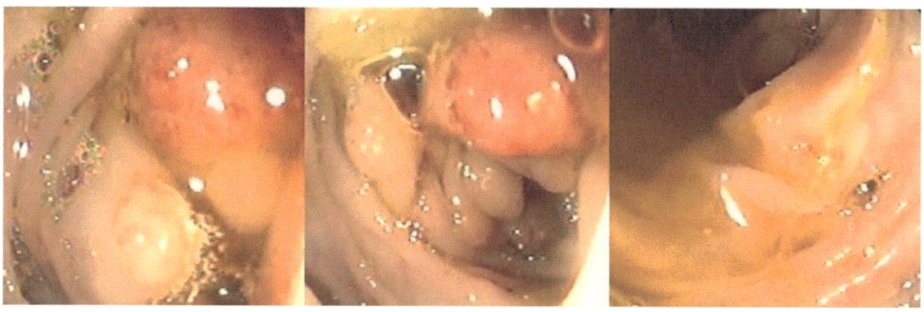

Figure 1.
Endoscopic appearance of a case of SCAD. A large, swollen, and red lesion on the top of the colonic fold can be seen: This lesion could be scored as type A SCAD.

9. Classification

SCAD can be classified endoscopically into four categories considering the absence of diverticulitis (**Table 1**) [3, 12, 14, 18, 19]:

The feature that unifies the four types of SCAD is the fact that it saves diverticular orifice. The main points used to classify SCAD in the different categories are how much it resembles or does not have mild-to-moderate UC, severe UC, or CD [12].

In the figures below, taken from Tursi, 2010, we observe endoscopic and histopathological images of SCAD type A (**Figure 2**), SCAD type B (**Figure 3**), SCAD type C (**Figure 4**), and SCAD type D (**Figure 5**) [2].

Type	Pattern	Endoscopic appearance	Histological appearance
A	**Crescentic fold**	Swollen red patches as of 0.5 to 1.5 cm in diameter.	Without architectural changes in the crypts. Neutrophil and lymphocyte infiltrate are limited to crypt epithelium.
B	**Mild to moderate UC-like**	Diffuse loss of vascular pattern, mucosal edema and hyperemia, and diffuse erosions.	Active inflammation with architectural changes in the crypt, crypt abscesses, and goblet cell depletion. Chronic changes of the lamina propria.
C	**Crohn's colitis-like**	Isolated aphthous ulcers.	Highest variability. Transmural inflammation with microfissures. Lymphoid follicles and non-specific infiltrates.
D	**Severe UC-like**	As type B but more severe with diffuse ulceration and reduced caliber of the lumen.	Crypt architectural changes, diffuse cryptitis, crypt abscesses, and goblet cell depletion. Chronic changes of the lamina propria.

Table 1.
SCAD classification (endoscopic and histological appearance).

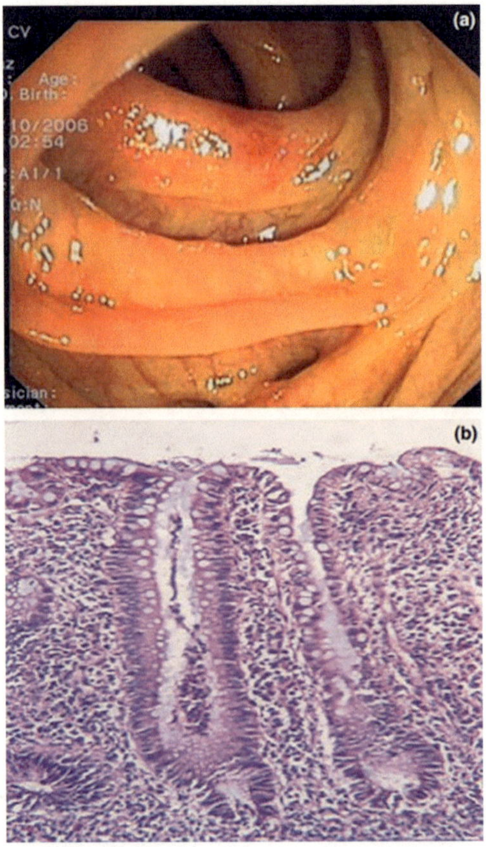

Figure 2.
Segmental colitis associated with diverticulosis' as "crescentic fold disease." The endoscopic pattern shows a swollen red patch about 1 cm in diameter, without hemorrhage or ulceration, confined to the crescentic mucosal fold. The diverticular orifices are spared, as well as the vascular pattern of the colonic mucosa is spared (a). The histopathological pattern shows an acute-on-chronic inflammation. Two crypt abscesses are evident in the center of the field (Hematoxylin & Eosin, magnification x20) (b).

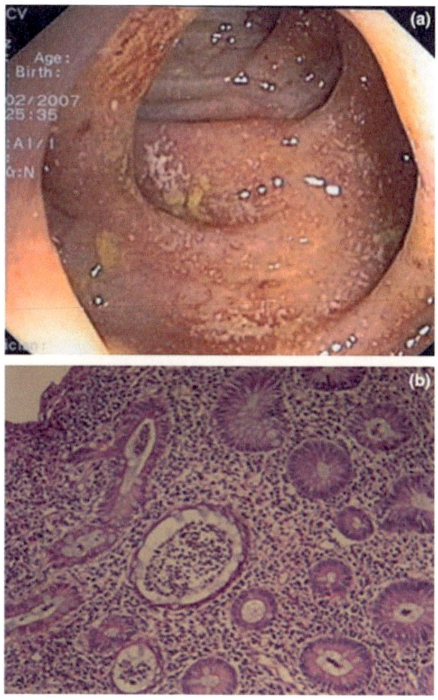

Figure 3.
Segmental colitis associated with diverticulosis as "Mild-to-moderate ulcerative colitis-like." the endoscopic pattern shows patchy loss of vascular pattern, edema, and hyperemia of the mucosa, and diffuse erosions. All diverticular orifices are spared (a). The histopathological pattern shows an acute-on-chronic inflammation. Two crypt abscesses are evident in the center of the field. There is also slight disarray and an architectural distortion with crypts irregularly arranged and varying in size and shape, patchy lymphoplasmacytic inflammation with some eosinophils (Hematoxylin & Eosin, magnification x100) (b).

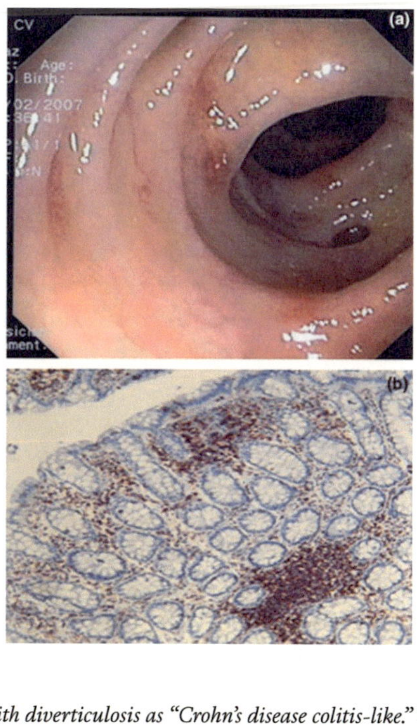

Figure 4.
Segmental colitis associated with diverticulosis as "Crohn's disease colitis-like." The endoscopic pattern shows scattered aphthous ulcers, some of them on the crescentic mucosal fold, within a normal colonic mucosa, with the normal vascular pattern. The diverticular orifices are always spared (a). The histopathological pattern shows a patchy lymphoplasmacytic inflammation in the upper part of the field, without significant cryptic architectural changes, and with a lymphoid follicle (count lymphocyte assay, magnification x20) (b).

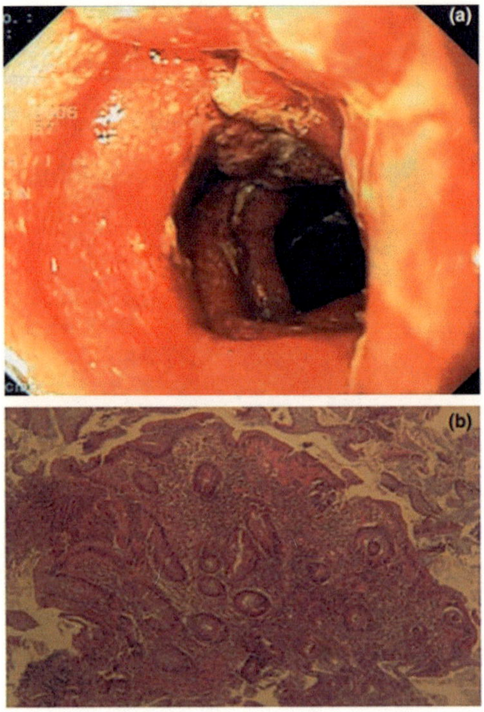

Figure 5.
Segmental colitis associated with diverticulosis as "Severe ulcerative colitis-like" SCAD pattern. The endoscopic pattern shows marked edema in the sigmoid mucosa with ulcerations, reduction of the lumen, diffuse loss of vascular pattern, diffuse hyperemia, and easy bleeding on contact with colonoscopy. The diverticular orifices are not easy to recognize, but they may be visible, spared by inflammation, at the maximal air inflation (a). Histology showed severe active ulcerative colitis (indistinguishable from classic inflammatory bowel disease), with severe diffuse inflammatory infiltrate, crypts irregularly arranged with architectural distortion, and cryptic abscesses (Hematoxylin & Eosin, magnification x40) (b).

10. Treatment

Since SCAD can resemble inflammatory diseases. It could be treated following the precepts of mild forms of IBD [3]. It is considered more benign than other IBD, with some patients evolving with full resolution of the condition without recurrences, even without any type of treatment being established [4, 10]. Types A and C SCAD seem to show a milder evolution, while types B and D have a high propensity to relapse, being highly indicated a more aggressive clinical and endoscopic follow-up and treatment for these two types [12, 20].

The standard treatment for SCAD is still not well defined, and it is possible to use a high fiber diet, use antibiotics (e.g., ciprofloxacin 500 mg twice a day associated with metronidazole 500 mg three times a day for 7 days) and aminosalicylates (mesalamine 2.4 to 3.2 g per day) in cases of unsatisfactory response to antibiotics or recurrent symptoms, which can be continued for 7 to 10 days or have its dose increased in case of therapeutic failure [4, 10, 14]. Immunosuppressants and steroids are used in severe third-line cases [4, 10].

In case of recurrence after having responded to the use of antibiotic therapy, we suggest repeating the same regimen for a long time.

Recent studies have demonstrated the possibility of combining beclomethasone dipropionate (BDP) (for 4 weeks) and the probiotic VSL#3 (for 15 days in a row) for the treatment of mild-to-moderate acute conditions, with the vast majority of patients reaching remission in week 4 [4, 10].

In patients' refractory to conventional therapy for SCAD, infliximab and adalimumab could be good therapeutic options [5, 21–23].

Table 2 shows the medicament advice, posology, and suggested time of use.

Surgery reserved for cases refractory to clinical treatment or that become dependent on corticosteroid therapy [4, 10].

It is always important to rethink whether the SCAD diagnosis is correct in case of failure of the instituted therapies, always bearing in mind the differential diagnoses, especially IBD [22].

The treatment algorithm for SCAD adapted from Kucej and Poggio 2018 is shown in **Figure 6** and divides the therapeutic indications according to the SCAD classification [3].

Medicament	Posology	Usage time
Ciprofloxacin	500 mg twice a day	7–14 days
metronidazole	500 mg 3 times a day	7–14 days
Mesalamine	2.4 a 3.2 g per day	Variable with the answer
Prednisone	40 mg + wean	7 days + weaning until week 6
Beclomethasone dipropionate	10 mg/day (1 month) + 5 mg/day (next month)	8 weeks
VSL#3	1 bag/day	15 days

Table 2.
Medicament, posology, and usage time for SCAD.

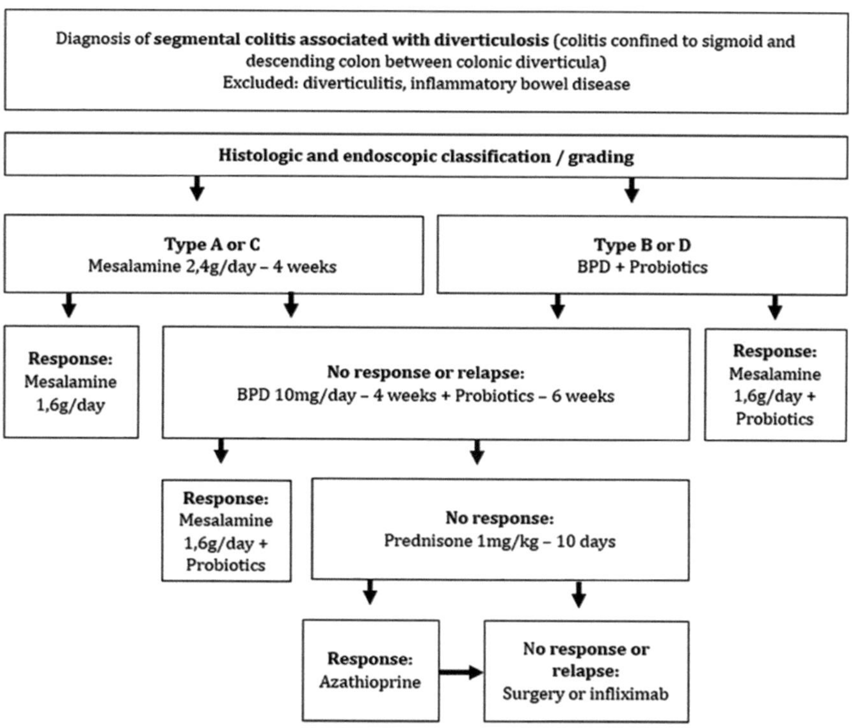

Figure 6.
Proposed algorithm for SCAD management (adapted by Tursi et al. [2]).

Conflict of interest

The authors declare no conflict of interest.

Abbreviations

SCAD	Segmental colitis associated with diverticulosis
IBD	Inflammatory bowel diseases
CD	Crohn's disease
UC	Ulcerative colitis

Author details

Rafael Luís Luporini[1,2*], Marcel Domeniconi[2], Ana Carolina Parra[2], André Rizzo[2], Daniela Freitas[2], Sthefânia Frizol[2] and Antonio Tursi[3]

1 Department of Medicine, Federal University of São Carlos (UFSCar), São Paulo, Brazil

2 General Surgery of Santa Casa de São Carlos, São Paulo, Brazil

3 Territorial Gastroenterology Service, Azienda Sanitaria Locale BAT, Andria, Italy

*Address all correspondence to: rafaelluporini@ufscar.br

References

[1] Tursi A, Scarpignato C, Strate LL, Lanas A, Kruis W, Lahat A, et al. Colonic diverticular disease. Nature Reviews Disease Primers. 2020;**6**(1):20. Available from: http://www.nature.com/articles/s41572-020-0153-5

[2] Tursi A, Elisei W, Brandimarte G, Giorgetti GM, Lecca PG, Di Cesare L, et al. The endoscopic spectrum of segmental colitis associated with diverticulosis. Colorectal Disease. 2010;**12**(5):464-470

[3] Kucej RJ, Poggio JL. Considerations and changes in the evaluation, management, and outcomes in the management of diverticular disease: The diagnosis, pathology, and treatment of diverticular colitis. Clinics in Colon and Rectal Surgery. 2018;**31**(4):221-225

[4] Schembri J. Segmental colitis associated with diverticulosis: Is it the coexistence of colonic diverticulosis and inflammatory bowel disease? Annals of Gastroenterology. 2017;**30**(3):257-261. Available from: http://www.annalsgastro.gr/files/journals/1/earlyview/2017/ev-01-2017-07-AG2943-0126.pdf

[5] Ghalyaie N. Management of diverticular disease in the setting of other colorectal pathology: Data on simultaneous issues in segmental colitis, inflammatory bowel disease, cancer, and complications. Clinics in Colon and Rectal Surgery. 2018;**31**(04):226-228. Available from: http://www.thieme-connect.de/DOI/DOI?10.1055/s-0037-1607468

[6] Tursi A. Segmental colitis associated with diverticulosis: Complication of diverticular disease or autonomous entity? Digestive Diseases and Sciences. 2011;**56**(1):27-34

[7] Lanas A, Abad-Baroja D, Lanas-Gimeno A. Progress and challenges in the management of diverticular disease: Which treatment? Therapeutic Advances in Gastroenterology. 2018;**11**: 175628481878905. Available from: http://journals.sagepub.com/doi/10.1177/1756284818789055

[8] Mărginean CO, Meliț LE, Mărginean MO. Segmental colitis associated diverticulosis-A possible diagnosis in teenagers. Frontiers in Pediatrics. 2018;**6**(June):1-5

[9] Freeman HJ. Segmental colitis associated diverticulosis syndrome. World Journal of Gastroenterology. 2016;**22**(36):8067-8069

[10] Piscopo N, Ellul P. Diverticular disease: A review on pathophysiology and recent evidence. The Ulster Medical Journal. 2020;**89**(2):83-88. Available from http://www.ncbi.nlm.nih.gov/pubmed/33093692

[11] Ludeman L, Shepherd NA. What is diverticular colitis? Pathology. 2002;**34**(6):568-572

[12] Schembri J, Bonello J, Christodoulou DK, Katsanos KH, Ellul P. Segmental colitis associated with diverticulosis: Is it the coexistence of colonic diverticulosis and inflammatory bowel disease? Annals of Gastroenterology. 2017;**30**(3):257-261

[13] Tursi A, Elisei W, Giorgetti G, Aiello F, Brandimarte G. Role of fecal calprotectin in the diagnosis and treatment of segmental colitis associated with diverticulosis. Minerva Gastroenterologica e Dietologica. 2011;**57**(3):247-255. Available from http://www.ncbi.nlm.nih.gov/pubmed/21769075

[14] Pemberton J et al. Segmental colitis associated with diverticulosis. In: Ted. W. Post, ed. UpToDate. Waltham, MA:

UpToDate; 2020. https://www.uptodate.com/contents/segmental-colitis-associated-with-diverticulosis?search=Segmental colitis associated with diverticulosis &source=search_result&selectedTitle=1~3&usage_type=default&display_rank=1. Accessed August 21, 2021.

[15] Hale WB. Colonoscopy in the diagnosis and management of diverticular disease. Journal of Clinical Gastroenterology. 2008 Nov;**42**(10):1142-1144. Available from: https://journals.lww.com/00004836-200811000-00024

[16] Tursi A, Brandimarte G, Elisei W, Giorgetti GM, Inchingolo CD, Danese S, et al. Assessment and grading of mucosal inflammation in colonic diverticular disease. Journal of Clinical Gastroenterology. 2008;**42**(6):699-703

[17] Goldstein NS, Leon-Armin C, Mani A. Crohn's colitis-like changes in sigmoid diverticulitis specimens is usually an idiosyncratic inflammatory response to the diverticulosis rather than Crohn's colitis. American Journal of Surgical Pathology. 2000;**24**(5):668-675

[18] Tursi A, Elisei W, Giorgetti GM, Inchingolo CD, Nenna R, Picchio M, et al. Segmental colitis associated with diverticulosis: A 5-year follow-up. International Journal of Colorectal Disease. 2012;**27**(2):179-185

[19] Al-Obaid L, McCarty TR, Bazarbashi AN, Wieczorek TJ, Rangel E, Homenko D. Segmental colitis associated with diverticulosis causing hydroureteronephrosis. ACG Case Reports Journal. 2019;**6**(11): e00253

[20] Tursi A, Elisei W, Giorgetti GM, Aiello F, Brandimarte G. Inflammatory manifestations at colonoscopy in patients with colonic diverticular disease. Alimentary Pharmacology and Therapeutics. 2011;**33**(3):358-365

[21] Hassan C. Tumour necrosis factor downregulation and therapeutic response to infliximab in a case of segmental colitis associated with diverticula. Gut. 2006;**55**(4):589-590. Available from: https://gut.bmj.com/lookup/doi/10.1136/gut.2005.084756

[22] Cassieri C, Brandimarte G, Elisei W, Lecca GP, Goni E, Penna A, et al. How to differentiate segmental colitis associated with diverticulosis and inflammatory bowel diseases. Journal of Clinical Gastroenterology. 2016;**50**(October): S36-S38

[23] Tursi A, Nenna R, Danese S. Therapeutic response to adalimumab in a case of steroid-dependent segmental colitis associated with diverticulosis. American Journal of Gastroenterology. 2021;**116**(8):1760-1761. DOI:10.14309/ajg.0000000000001226

Section 3

Complicated Colonic Diverticular Disease

Chapter 3

Complicated Colonic Diverticular Disease – Diagnostic and Therapeutic Difficulties

Cristian Mesina, Theodor Viorel Dumitrescu, Mihai Calin Ciorbagiu, Cosmin Vasile Obleaga and Mihaela-Iustina Mesina Botoran

Abstract

Diverticular disease is one of the most common problems encountered by general surgeons and gastroenterologists. The term refers to complications that occur from colonic diverticulosis. In diverticular colonic disease the sigmoid colon is usually the most commonly involved, while right acute colonic diverticulitis is rarer. In establishing the diagnosis of ALCD, objective clinical examination plays an important role in addition to biological paraclinical examinations (C-reactive protein - CRP and increased leukocyte count) and radiological paraclinical examinations: CT abdomen. CRP is a useful tool in predicting the clinical severity of acute diverticulitis. The treatment applied to patients with uncomplicated colonic diverticular disease can be represented by antibiotic therapy, water regime, hydro-electrolytic rebalancing. In patients with multiple comorbidities, hemodynamic instability, the Hartmann procedure is recommended for the treatment of acute peritonitis caused by perforated colonic diverticulitis and in hemodynamically stable patients without comorbidities, colonic resection with primary anastomosis with or without stoma is suggested.

Keywords: acute left colonic diverticulosis, acute right colonic diverticulitis, hartmann segmental colectomy, hemorrhagic colonic diverticulosis, perforating diverticular disease, acute fistulized diverticulitis

1. Introduction

Diverticular disease is one of the most common problems encountered by general surgeons and gastroenterologists. The term refers to complications that occur from colonic diverticulosis, including lower gastrointestinal bleeding, inflammation, pain, abscess formation, fistula, strictures, perforation, and death [1]. It is an important cause of morbidity and a significant economic burden [1, 2]. Acute left colonic diverticulosis is common in Western countries, with its prevalence increasing worldwide, which is probably due to lifestyle changes [1]. Although left colonic diverticulosis remains more common in elderly patients, a dramatic increase in its incidence has been observed in younger age groups in recent years [2]. Recent evidence suggests that the risk of developing acute left colonic diverticulitis (ALCD)

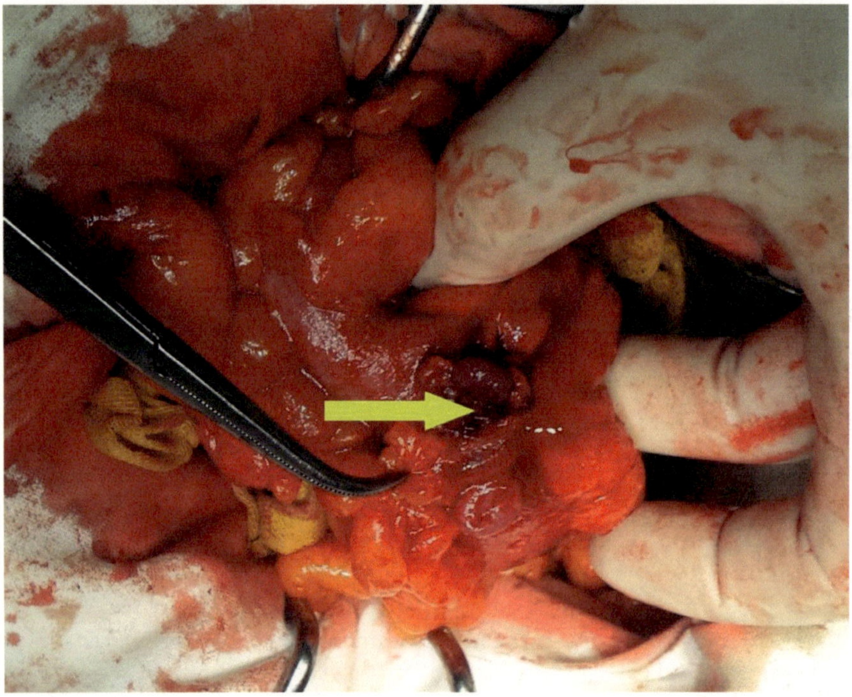

Figure 1.
Intraoperative demonstration of the colo-bladder fistula. Surgical examination of the pelvic peritoneal cavity showed a colo-bladder fistula with a diameter of 0.4 cm (yellow arrow).

for life is approximately 4% in patients with diverticulosis [3], and data from Western populations suggest that up to one-fifth of patients with acute diverticulitis have less than 50 years of age [4–6]. ALCD is a common problem encountered by Western surgeons in the acute context. The sigmoid colon is usually the most commonly involved, while right acute colonic diverticulitis (ARCD) is rarer, but much more common in non-Western populations. A diagnosis of diverticular disease should not be overlooked in younger patients, as hospitalization rates in those under the age of 40 have increased significantly in the last decade. In most cases, uncomplicated acute diverticulitis can be treated medically with antibiotics and digestive rest or with a clear liquid diet. Uncomplicated acute diverticulitis can be managed on an outpatient basis in selected patients who do not have comorbidities (including the immunocompromised state) and can tolerate a liquid diet in the absence of fever, significant leukocytosis, or evidence of complicated imaging disease. Recurrent diverticulitis or diverticulitis complications, including abscess, perforation, fistulizing disease (**Figure 1**), and strictures/obstruction usually require surgery.

2. Classification of colonic diverticular disease

In 2016, the guidelines of the World Society of Emergency Surgery (WSES) were published [7], and in 2020 the guidelines were revised in accordance with the GRADE methodology [8, 9]. The GRADE system is a hierarchical evidence-based tool that systematically evaluates the available literature. Following the study of the available literature, it was concluded that there are several classification systems for ALCD. Hinchey and colleagues rated the severity of acute diverticulitis at 4 degrees [10] in patients with clinical findings of intra-abdominal abscesses:

1. Abscess around the colon

2. Pelvic, intra-abdominal or retroperitoneal abscess

3. Generalized purulent peritonitis

4. Generalized fecal peritonitis

In recent years, computed tomography (CT) has become a diagnostic tool in the staging of patients with ALCD, so the Hinchey classification has been changed [11–15]. Thus, Neff et al. [11] presented a new classification in 5 stages, from stage 0 (uncomplicated) to stage 4 (pneumoperitoneum with abundant free fluid in the peritoneal cavity).

0 - Uncomplicated diverticulitis; diverticula, thickening of the wall, increased density of pericolic fat
1 - Complicated local with local abscess
2 - Complicated with pelvic abscess
3 - Complicated with distant abscess
4 - Complicated with other complications at a distance

In 2002, Ambrosetti et al. [12] classified ALCD as moderate disease and severe disease based on CT examination. Moderate diverticulitis was defined by thickening of the colon walls ≥5 mm and signs of inflammation of the fat around the affected colon and severe diverticulitis was defined by thickening of the colon walls, accompanied by abscess, extraluminal gas or extraluminal contrast substance:

1. Moderate diverticulitis

   a. Thickening of the wall of the localized sigmoid colon (≥ 5 mm)

   b. Infiltration of fat around the colon

2. Severe diverticulitis

   a. Abscess

   b. Extraluminal gas

   c. Extraluminal contrast

In 2005, Kaiser and colleagues [13] modified the Hinchey classification in accordance with the CT examination. Thus diverticulitis was classified into 5 stages:

Stage 0: mild clinical form diverticulitis
Stage 1a: limited inflammation around the colon
Stage 1b: limited abscess around the colon
Stage 2: pelvic or distal intra-abdominal abscess
Stage 3: generalized purulent peritonitis
Stage 4: fecal peritonitis at presentation

Mora Lopez and co-workers [14] in 2013 proposed a change to the Neff classification by dividing stage 1 of the Neff classification into:

- stage 1a - pneumoperitoneum located in the form of gas bubbles
- stage 1b - abscess <4 cm

The Mora Lopez classification is as follows:

- stage 0 - uncomplicated diverticulitis: colonic diverticulum, thickening of the colon wall, increased density of fat around the colon
- stage 1 - locally complicated diverticulitis:
  - 1a Pneumoperitoneum located in the form of gas bubbles
  - 1b Abscess (<4 cm)
- stage 2 - complicated diverticulitis with pelvic abscess. Abscess>4 cm in the pelvis
- stage 3 - complicated diverticulitis with distant abscess. Abscess in the abdominal cavity (outside the pelvis)
- stage 4 - complicated diverticulitis with other distant complications. Abundant pneumoperitoneum and / or free intra-abdominal fluid

Sallinen et al. [15] conducted a retrospective study on patients treated for ALCD and established the following staging:

stage 1 - Uncomplicated diverticulitis
stage 2 - Complicated diverticulitis with small abscess (<6 cm)
stage 3 - Complicated diverticulitis with large abscess (≥ 6 cm) or distant intraperitoneal or retroperitoneal gas
stage 4 - Generalized peritonitis without organ dysfunction
stage 5 - Generalized peritonitis with organ dysfunction

In 2015, the WSES study group [16] proposed a classification of ALCD based on CT examination of the abdomen:

- uncomplicated diverticulitis: thickening of the colon wall, increasing the density of fat around the colon
- complicated diverticulitis which is divided into 4 stages depending on the extent of the infectious process:

Stage 1

1A Air bubbles around the affected colon or small amount of fluid around the colon without abscess (5 cm from the inflamed intestinal segment).
1B Abscess ≤4 cm

Stage 2

2A Abscess>4 cm
2B Gas at a distance (> 5 cm from the inflamed intestinal segment)

Stage 3 - Diffuse fluid without free gas at a distance
Stage 4 - Diffuse fluid with free gas at a distance

3. Establishing the diagnosis of acute diverticulitis

In establishing the diagnosis of ALCD, objective clinical examination plays an important role in addition to biological paraclinical examinations (C-reactive protein - CRP and increased leukocyte count) and radiological paraclinical examinations: CT abdomen. CRP has been identified as a useful biomarker of inflammation and may be useful in predicting the clinical severity of acute diverticulitis, as demonstrated by several recent studies [17–19]. To investigate the value of CRP and other laboratory parameters of patients in predicting the clinical severity of acute diverticulitis, a retrospective study was published in 2014 [17]. The authors concluded that CRP is a useful tool in predicting the clinical severity of acute diverticulitis. A mild episode is very likely in patients with CRP less than 170 mg/l. Those with higher CRP values are more likely to undergo surgery or percutaneous drainage.

Mäkelä and colleagues [19] published a study comparing CRP values in 350 patients who first experienced symptoms of acute diverticulitis with CT results and clinical parameters, both by univariate and multivariate analyzes. The CRP limit value of 149.5 mg / l significantly discriminated uncomplicated acute diverticulitis from complicated diverticulitis (specificity 65%, sensitivity 85%, area under curve 0.811, p = 0.0001). In the multivariate analysis, a CRP value above 150 mg/l and advanced age were independent risk factors for complicated acute diverticulitis. The mean CRP was significantly higher in deceased patients (mean CRP of 207 mg/l) than in those who survived (mean CRP of 139 mg/l). In addition, a CRP value above

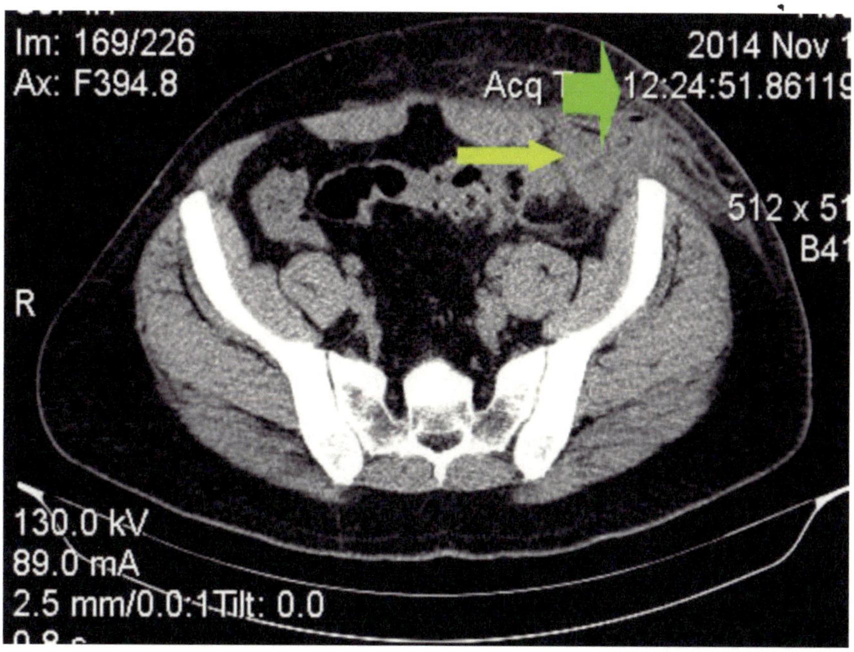

Figure 2.
CT abdomen and pelvis in a patient with colonic diverticulosis complicated by colo-cutaneous fistula: the presence of a fluid collection and areas of air bubbles in the muscles of the abdominal wall (green arrow) and the disappearance of the cleavage plane of the small intestine (yellow arrow).

150 mg/l and free abdominal fluid in CT were independent variables that predicted postoperative mortality. The study confirmed that CRP is useful for predicting the severity of acute diverticulitis on admission. The authors concluded that patients with a CRP value greater than 150 mg/l have an increased risk of complicated diverticulitis and should always undergo a CT scan.

CT abdomen with contrast agent is the radiological examination that is used to evaluate patients with suspected ALCD. This approach is the gold standard for both diagnosis and staging of patients with ALCD due to its excellent sensitivity and specificity [20–22]. CT can also rule out other diagnoses, such as ovarian pathology or abdominal aortic aneurysm. CT findings in patients with ALCD may include diverticulosis with associated colonic wall thickening, increased fat density around the affected colon, extraluminal gas, pneumoperitoneum, abscess formation, or free intra-abdominal fluid (**Figure 2**).

4. Acute diverticulitis: treatment

4.1 ALCD in immunocompromised patients

Immunocompromised patients have an increased risk of complicated ALCD [23–26]. As such, most of these patients require urgent surgery, and this is associated with a significantly higher mortality rate [27]. A recent study by Biondo et al. [28] analyzed the relationship between the different causes of immunosuppression (IMS) and ALCD. Immunocompromised patients were divided into 5 groups according to the causes of IMS: group I, chronic corticosteroids; group II, transplant patients; group III, malignant neoplasm disease; group IV, chronic renal failure; and group V, other immunosuppressive treatments. The rate of emergency surgery was high (39.3%) and was required more frequently in group I (chronic corticosteroid therapy). In this study, postoperative mortality was 31.6%, and the recurrence rate after a successful non-operative control occurred in 30 patients (27.8%).

4.2 Antibiotic treatment in patients with uncomplicated acute colonic diverticulitis

Uncomplicated acute diverticulitis is an intra-abdominal infection in which the infectious process does not extend beyond the affected colon, while in complicated acute diverticulitis the infectious process extends beyond the colon, producing either localized peritonitis or diffuse peritonitis [29]. Studies have been done on the use of antibiotics in uncomplicated acute diverticulitis. A multicenter study published by Chabok and colleagues in 2012 [30], performed in surgical clinics in Sweden and Iceland on 623 patients with uncomplicated acute diverticulitis confirmed by CT examination, showed that antibiotic treatment applied to uncomplicated acute diverticulitis did not lead to a more accelerated cure of the disease nor to the prevention of complications or recurrence of the disease.

Therefore, antibiotic treatment for uncomplicated acute diverticulitis is not indicated and antibiotics should be reserved for complicated acute diverticulitis only. However, the high mortality associated with sepsis requires the clinician to maintain a high index of clinical suspicion in patients who are prone to an increased risk of sepsis [31]. Thus, in patients with uncomplicated acute diverticulitis confirmed by CT examination, having an increased risk of sepsis such as patients with clinical manifestations of infection or in elderly patients, immunocompromised or with comorbidities that decrease the immune response, spectrum antibiotic therapy is suggested. Must cover gram-negative and anaerobic bacilli.

In 2009, a randomized controlled trial of oral antibiotic therapy versus intravenous antibiotic therapy (ciprofloxacin and metronidazole) was performed for patients with uncomplicated acute diverticulitis [32]. Intravenous antibiotic therapy has not been shown to be more effective than oral antibiotic therapy in uncomplicated acute diverticulitis. For patients with uncomplicated ALCD and without comorbidities, it is suggested that treatment be performed in a specialty outpatient setting. It is necessary to re-evaluate at 7 days, and if the clinical condition deteriorates, the re-evaluation must be done earlier and the patients with significant comorbidities who have vomiting, the hydro-electrolytic rebalancing will be done by hospitalization.

4.3 Treatment of patients with uncomplicated ALCD

Etzioni et al. [33] published a retrospective study in 2010, showing that outpatient treatment was effective for 94% of patients with acute diverticulitis. A systematic review of the outpatient management of uncomplicated acute diverticulitis has recently been published [34]. Jackson et al. concluded that current evidence suggested that outpatient treatment for most cases of uncomplicated acute diverticulitis was warranted. Rodríguez-Cerrillo et al. [35] have recently shown that elderly patients with comorbidities can also be treated safely at home, avoiding hospitalization. The DIVER trial [36] demonstrated that outpatient treatment can be safe and effective in selected patients with uncomplicated acute diverticulitis without comorbidities and can reduce costs without negatively affecting the quality of life of these patients. This multicenter study included patients over 18 years of age with uncomplicated acute diverticulitis. Confirmation of uncompleted acute diverticulitis was made by abdominal CT examination. The first dose of antibiotic was given intravenously to all patients in the emergency department, and then the patients were either hospitalized or discharged. Out of a total of 132 patients, treatment failure was recorded in 4 hospitalized patients and in 3 at home they developed treatment failure (there were no differences between groups ($p = 0.62$)). The overall cost of healthcare per episode was 3 times lower in the outpatient group, with significant cost savings of EUR 1124.70 per patient. No differences were observed between groups in terms of quality of life.

4.4 Treatment in patients with acute diverticulitis discovered on CT by the presence of gas around the colon

The best treatment in patients with complicated acute diverticulitis confirmed by CT examination that shows the presence of free gas around the affected colon, the WSES group recommends a non-operative treatment with antibiotic therapy [16]. Among patients hospitalized for acute diverticulitis, 15–25% of patients have an abscess around the affected colon, detected by CT examination [37]. When the size of the abscess around the affected colon is around 4–5 cm, an antibiotic treatment can be tried, but with a failure rate of 20% and a mortality rate of 0.6% [38]. Percutaneous drainage of the abscess combined with antibiotic treatment [39–43] is also discussed in these patients. Surgical treatment is required in these patients when they show clinical signs of sepsis. In 2015, a retrospective study was published by Elagili et al. [44] comparing antibiotic-only treatment of diverticular abscess versus percutaneous drainage. In this study, 32 patients were treated with antibiotics alone and 114 underwent percutaneous drainage. Surgery was required to remove the abscess in 8 patients who underwent antibiotic therapy alone (25%) and in 21 patients (18%) who underwent percutaneous drainage. In patients with percutaneous drainage, special attention should be paid to the drainage catheter.

Removal of this drainage catheter should be considered when the drainage flow has decreased significantly and on CT examination with contrast medium, no identifiable cavity remains around the catheter, in which case the catheter will be removed. If a decrease in the abscess is not noticed on the CT examination and the patient does not show any improvement in the clinical situation, the following therapeutic decisions may be necessary: additional drainage, repositioning of the drainage catheter or an abscess removal surgery.

In patients with acute diverticulitis with findings on CT examination, free gas at a distance without diffuse intra-abdominal fluid, a non-operative treatment is suggested, only if a careful and continuous monitoring of the patient can be performed. Of these patients, about 25% treated non-operatively may require emergency surgery [45]. If these patients show signs of acute peritonitis at the clinical examination, then emergency surgery, hydro-electrolytic rebalancing, antibiotic therapy are required. Dharmarajan et al. [46] reported a high success rate for nonoperative management in patients with acute diverticulitis and free gas on CT examination, but excluding those with hemodynamic instability. Sallinen et al. [47] concluded that non-operative treatment can be applied to patients with acute diverticulitis and distant free gas highlighted by CT examination, but in the absence of diffuse acute peritonitis or fluid in the bottom of the Douglas sac. The appearance of a massive pneumoperitoneum or the presence of gas in the retroperitoneal space even in the absence of generalized acute peritonitis, was associated with a non-operative treatment failure rate of 57–60%. Surgery in patients with clinical signs of acute peritonitis with acute perforated diverticulitis should be surgical resection of the affected colon and anastomosis with or without stoma, in stable patients without comorbidities and the Hartmann procedure (HP) in hemodynamically unstable patients or in patients with multiple comorbidities [16].

4.5 Follow-up of patients treated for colonic diverticular abscess

In patients with uncomplicated acute diverticulitis confirmed by non-operative CT examination, a routine assessment of the colon is not recommended, while in patients with non-operatively treated diverticular abscess an early assessment of the colon at 4–6 weeks is recommended. A perforated colon cancer with localized colon abscess, although less common but possible, may mimic acute colonic diverticulitis with abscess around the colon [48, 49]. It has been shown that the risk of malignancy after uncomplicated acute diverticulitis proven by CT is low, so that a routine colonoscopy, in the absence of other indications, is not necessary. In 2014, a study [50] was published investigating the rate of colorectal cancer (CRC) discovered by colonoscopy after an episode of uncomplicated diverticulitis. A total of 2,490 patients with uncomplicated diverticulitis were included in the study. 17 patients were diagnosed with CRC (1.16%). Hyperplastic polyps were observed in 156 patients (10.6%), low-grade adenoma in 90 patients (6.1%) and adenoma with aggravated dysplasia in 32 patients (2.2%). This study shows that routine colonoscopic evaluation in the absence of other clinical signs of CRC is not necessary in patients who have had an episode of uncomplicated acute diverticulitis.

4.6 Treatment of patients with acute peritonitis caused by perforated colonic diverticulitis

In patients with acute diffuse peritonitis due to diverticular perforation, lavage and laparoscopic drainage are suggested only in carefully selected patients. A minimally invasive approach using laparoscopic peritoneal lavage and drainage has been debated in recent years as an alternative to colon resection [51]. This therapeutic procedure consists of laparoscopic aspiration of the pus followed by copious washing of the peritoneal cavity and placement of abdominal drainage tubes, which remain many days after this procedure. In 2013, a retrospective Dutch analysis of 38 patients [52] with perforated acute colonic diverticulitis peritonitis was published. In 7 patients, this approach did not control sepsis, 2 patients died from multiple organ dysfunction syndrome (MODS) and 5 patients required additional surgery (3 Hartmann resections, 1 stoma and 1 perforation suture). Predictors for the failure of conservative therapy (drainage and laparoscopic lavage) were: multiple comorbidities, high CRP levels and a high Manheim index of peritonitis. In 2015, the results of the SCANDIV study were published [53]. According to this study, laparoscopic lavage is not supported for the treatment of acute perforated colonic diverticulitis. The LADIES study published in 2015 [54] showed that laparoscopic lavage was not superior to sigmoidectomy for the treatment of acute perforated diverticulitis. So in acute Hinchey III diverticulitis, laparoscopic lavage is marred by an increased failure rate with the need for reintervention for intra-abdominal abscess.

In patients with multiple comorbidities, hemodynamic instability, the Hartmann (HP) procedure is recommended for the treatment of acute peritonitis caused by perforated colonic diverticulitis and in hemodynamically stable patients without comorbidities, colonic resection with primary anastomosis with or without stoma is suggested. The HP is considered a therapeutic option in acute peritonitis caused by acute perforated colonic diverticulitis in patients presented in the emergency department with critical conditions and multiple comorbidities (**Figures 3** and **4**). However, restoration of intestinal transit continuity is associated with significant morbidity [55] and therefore many of these patients do not undergo digestive transit restoration surgery and thus remain with a permanent stoma [56]. A study that included 2729 patients [57] evaluated patients with acute perforated diverticulitis who were treated either by colon resection with primary anastomosis and protective ileostomy or by the HP. Most patients were treated by the HP and only 208 (7.6%) patients were treated by colon resection with primary anastomosis and protective ileostomy. Mortality rates for patients undergoing the HP and colon resection with the primary anastomosis were 7.6% and 2.9%, respectively. The authors concluded that colon resection with primary anastomosis and protective ileostomy may be the optimal therapeutic strategy for carefully selected patients with acute peritonitis caused by perforated colonic diverticulitis.

Oberkofler et al. [58] conducted a randomized colonic resection study in 2012 with primary anastomosis and protective ileostomy versus the HP in patients with

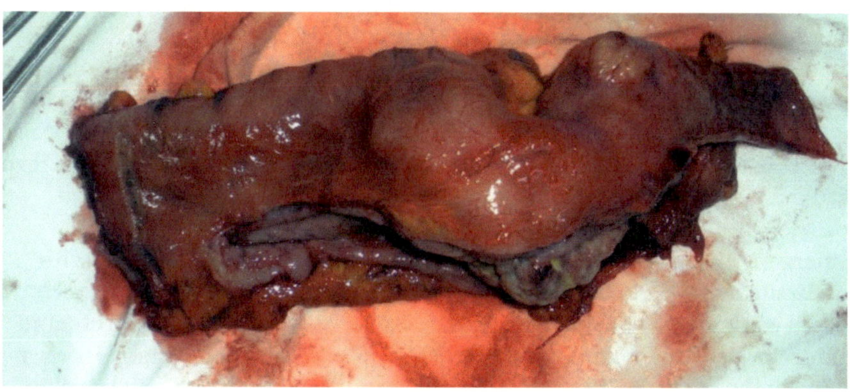

Figure 3.
Sigmoid colon resected in a patient with perforated sigmoid colonic diverticulosis.

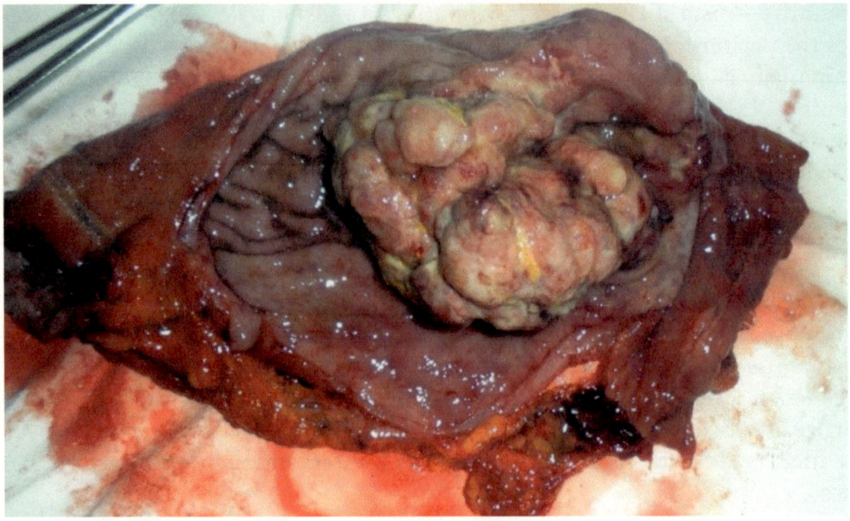

Figure 4.
Macroscopic appearance of a perforated sigmoid colonic diverticulosis on the sigmoidectomy resection piece.

acute peritonitis caused by perforated acute colonic diverticulitis. 62 patients with left colonic perforation (Hinchey III and IV) were randomized for the HP (30 patients) and for colon resection with primary anastomosis and protective ileostomy (32 patients). A planned operation to reintegrate the intestine into the digestive tract was performed at 3 months. The study did not report any difference in mortality and initial morbidity (mortality 13% vs. 9% and morbidity 67% vs. 75% in the HP versus colon resection with primary anastomosis), but found a reduction in hospital stay, lower costs, fewer serious complications in the colon resection group with primary anastomosis and protective ileostomy. The LADIES study [59] performed in 2019 in immunocompetent patients, hemodynamically stable, less than 85 years of age, showed that colon resection with primary anastomosis is preferable compared to the HP for the treatment of acute peritonitis by diverticulitis, acute perforated colon (Hinchey's disease III or IV). In this study were eligible patients aged 18 to 85 years who showed clinical signs of acute peritonitis caused by acute perforated colonic diverticulitis and CT abdomen showed free gas and fluid in the peritoneal cavity. Patients with Hinchey I or II diverticulitis were not eligible for inclusion.

A systematic review of the literature on the surgical management of Hinchey diverticulitis III and IV was published in 2019 [60]. 3596 patients were included in this study. Overall mortality in HP patients was 10.8% in observational studies, and at colon resection with primary anastomosis, mortality was lower, being 8.2% in observational studies.

4.7 The role of laparoscopic surgery in the treatment of diffuse acute peritonitis caused by acute perforated diverticulitis

Emergency laparoscopic sigmoidectomy is recommended in patients with diffuse acute peritonitis caused by perforated acute diverticulitis, only if technical skills and equipment are available. In 2015, a systematic review of laparoscopic sigmoidectomy in emergencies was published [61]. A total of 104 patients were included in the study: HP was performed in 84 patients and colon resection with primary anastomosis was performed in 20 patients. The average duration of hospitalization varied between 6 and 16 days, 3 patients died in the postoperative period.

This study showed that emergency laparoscopic sigmoidectomy is possible for the treatment of acute perforated sigmoid diverticulitis with generalized peritonitis, but laparoscopic sigmoidectomy was performed on selected patients and was performed in experienced centers. To demonstrate the benefits of laparoscopic sigmoidectomy compared to classic open surgery sigmoidectomy, high-quality prospective or randomized studies are needed.

4.8 Therapeutic strategy in diffuse acute peritonitis produced by acute perforated diverticulitis

Diffuse acute peritonitis caused by perforated acute colonic diverticulitis is a life-threatening condition that requires prompt emergency surgery. To improve the results, in recent years a treatment algorithm has been developed in patients with generalized acute peritonitis caused by acute perforated colonic diverticulitis, which consists of peritoneal lavage, segmental resection of the affected colon or closure of the perforation and the second surgery is performed at 3–6 months to restore bowel continuity [62, 63]. Patients who are hemodynamically unstable are not candidates for immediate complex surgery. Initial surgery in hemodynamically unstable patients with multiple comorbidities should be limited to controlling the source of peritoneal infection, for example primary closure of perforation / limited resection of the affected colon (HP) after which the patient is taken to the intensive care unit for rebalancing hydro-electrolytic, acid–base, correction of anemia, possibly correction of respiratory and circulatory deficits. In 2012, a prospective observational study was published by Kafka-Ritsah et al. [51]. In this study were enrolled 51 patients (28 women), with a mean age of 69 years with diverticulitis Hinchey III (40 patients - 78%) and Hinchey IV (11 patients - 22%). The hospitalized patients were initially treated by segmental resection of the affected colon, peritoneal lavage, followed by an operation at 24–48 hours to restore bowel continuity in 36 patients (84%), of which 4 patients underwent a protective ileostomy. There were 5 anastomotic fistulas. The overall mortality rate was 9.8%. WSES recommends using an open abdomen approach in selected patients with ongoing sepsis disorders [64]. In patients with ongoing severe sepsis, the open abdomen technique can be used with the application of therapy with negative active peritoneal pressure [65].

4.9 Factors considered for a segmental colonic resection in cases of non-operatively treated acute colonic diverticulitis

It is recommended that after an acute episode of ALCD conservatively treated, a segmental resection of the affected colon be performed, especially in immunocompromised patients. Older clinical trials have reported that about one-third of patients with acute diverticulitis will have a recurrent attack, often within 1 year [66, 67]. After a 4-year follow-up, El Sayed et al. [68] on an English study of 65,000 patients treated non-operatively for the first episode of acute colonic diverticulitis, found a recurrence rate of approximately 11.2%. The DIRECT, multicenter randomized trial was performed on 109 patients, performed on 26 hospitals in the Netherlands. Patients in the study had persistent and recurrent abdominal pain after an episode of acute colonic diverticulitis [69]. After this 6-month follow-up, the sigmoidectomy performed led to a better quality of life compared to non-operative management, evaluation performed through several specific questionnaires. Currently, the decision to segmental colectomy of the colon, performed after one or more episodes of acute colonic diverticulitis, must be made on a case-by-case basis taking into account risk factors, complications, age, severity of recurrent episodes, personal pathological history and comorbidities. (e.g. immunosuppressed patients) [70].

4.10 Duration of optimal antibiotic therapy after surgical control of the source of sepsis in acute peritonitis caused by acute perforated colonic diverticulitis

It is suggested a duration of 4 days of postoperative treatment with antibiotics in complicated ALCD if the source of peritoneal infection has been surgically suppressed. The therapeutic regimen should depend on the severity of the infection, the pathogens suspected to be involved and the risk factors for developing antibiotic resistance [28]. The pathogens involved are Gram-negative and Gram-positive bacteria as well as anaerobic bacteria. The main threat of resistance in intra-abdominal infections is Enterobactericeae which produce extended spectrum beta-lactamase (ESBL) which is becoming more common in community-acquired infections worldwide [71]. The recent study by Sawyer et al. [72] showed that in patients with intra-abdominal infections, the results of antibiotic treatment with a duration of 4 days were similar to those with a longer duration of antibiotic treatment.

4.11 Principles of treatment of right acute colonic diverticulitis (ARCD)

The principles of diagnosis and treatment of patients with ARCD are similar to those of patients with ALCD, although studies have shown that the percentage of complications requiring surgery is higher in patients with ALCD than in patients with ARCD. Typically, the sigmoid colon is more involved in acute colonic diverticulitis than the right colon - ARCD [73]. ARCD has a lower rate of complicated diverticulitis [74] and ARCD occurs more frequently in middle-aged men. In particular, ARCD is located on the cecum, making differential diagnosis with acute appendicitis difficult. CT abdomen with contrast agent has an essential role in establishing the diagnosis of ARCD [75]. The diagnostic and treatment principles of ARCD are similar to those of ALCD. As a therapeutic option in ARCD, non-operative methods should be preferred in cases without acute diffuse peritonitis, although differentiation from malignant proliferative processes is difficult [76]. Surgical treatment is usually performed in cases of complicated ARCD [73, 77–79]. In experienced medical centers, laparoscopic resection of the affected colon with primary anastomosis can be performed [80, 81].

5. Conclusions

1. In diverticular colonic disease the sigmoid colon is usually the most commonly involved, while right acute colonic diverticulitis is rarer.

2. In establishing the diagnosis of ALCD, objective clinical examination plays an important role in addition to biological paraclinical examinations (C-reactive protein - CRP and increased leukocyte count) and radiological paraclinical examinations: CT abdomen. CRP is a useful tool in predicting the clinical severity of acute diverticulitis.

3. CT abdomen with contrast agent is the radiological examination that is used to evaluate patients with suspected ALCD. This approach is the gold standard for both diagnosis and staging of patients with ALCD due to its excellent sensitivity and specificity.

4. In patients with acute diverticulitis with findings on CT examination, free gas at a distance without diffuse intra-abdominal fluid, a non-operative

treatment is suggested, only if a careful and continuous monitoring of the patient can be performed.

5. The treatment applied to patients with uncomplicated colonic diverticular disease can be represented by antibiotic therapy, water regime, hydro-electrolytic rebalancing.

6. In patients with multiple comorbidities, hemodynamic instability, the Hartmann procedure is recommended for the treatment of acute peritonitis caused by perforated colonic diverticulitis and in hemodynamically stable patients without comorbidities, colonic resection with primary anastomosis with or without stoma is suggested.

7. In patients with uncomplicated acute diverticulitis confirmed by non-operative CT examination, a routine assessment of the colon is not recommended, while in patients with non-operatively treated diverticular abscess an early assessment of the colon at 4–6 weeks is recommended.

8. Emergency laparoscopic sigmoidectomy is recommended in patients with diffuse acute peritonitis caused by perforated acute diverticulitis, only if technical skills and equipment are available.

9. In patients with acute diffuse peritonitis due to diverticular perforation, lavage and laparoscopic drainage are suggested only in carefully selected patients.

10. The principles of diagnosis and treatment of patients with ARCD are similar to those of patients with ALCD, although studies have shown that the percentage of complications requiring surgery is higher in patients with ALCD than in patients with ARCD.

Conflict of interest

The authors declare no conflict of interest.

Abbreviations

ARCD	Acute right colonic diverticulitis
ALCD	Acute left colonic diverticulitis
CT	Computed Tomography
CRP	C-reactive protein
CRC	Colorectal Cancer
ESBL	Extended Spectrum beta-lactamase
HP	Hartmann Procedure
IMS	Immunosuppression
MODS	Multiple Organ Dysfunction Syndrome
WSES	World Society of Emergency Surgery

Author details

Cristian Mesina[1*], Theodor Viorel Dumitrescu[1], Mihai Calin Ciorbagiu[1], Cosmin Vasile Obleaga[1] and Mihaela-Iustina Mesina Botoran[2]

1 Department of Surgery, Emergency County Hospital of Craiova, University of Medicine and Pharmacy of Craiova, Craiova, Romania

2 Department of Human Anatomy, University of Medicine and Pharmacy of Craiova, Craiova, Romania

*Address all correspondence to: mesina.cristian@doctor.com

References

[1] Rodky GV, Welch CE. Changing patterns in the surgical treatment of diverticular disease. Annals of surgery. 1984;**200**:466-478.

[2] Etzioni DA, Mack TM, Beart RW, et al. Diverticulisis in the United States: 1998-2005: Changing patterns of disease and treatment. Annals of surgery. 2009;**249**:210-217.

[3] Kozak LJ, DeFrances CJ, Hall MJ. National hospital discharge survery: 2004 annual summary with detailed diagnosis and procedure data. Vital and health statistics. 2006;**13**:1-209.

[4] Sandler RS, Everhart JE, Donowitz M, et al. The burden of selected digestive diseases in the United States. Gastroenterology. 2002;**122**: 1500-1511.

[5] Warner E, Crighton EJ, Moineddin R, et al. Fourteen-year study of hospital admissions for diverticular disease in Ontario. Canadian journal of gastroenterology. 2007;**21**:97-99.

[6] Painter NS, Burkitt DP. Diverituclar disease of the colon: A deficiency disease of Western civilization. British medical journal. 1971;**2**:450-454.

[7] Sartelli M, Catena F, Ansaloni L, Coccolini F, Griffiths EA, Abu-Zidan FM, et al. WSES guidelines for the management of acute left sided colonic diverticulitis in the emergency setting. World journal of emergency surgery. 2016;**11**:37.

[8] Guyatt GH, Oxman AD, Vist GE, Kunz R, Falck-Ytter Y, Alonso-Coello P, et al. GRADE: an emerging consensus on rating quality of evidence and strength of recommendations. British medical journal. 2008;**336**:924-926.

[9] Brozek JL, Akl EA, Jaeschke R, Lang DM, Bossuyt P, Glasziou P, et al. Grading quality of evidence and strength of recommendations in clinical practice guidelines: part 2 of 3. The GRADE approach to grading quality of evidence about diagnostic tests and strategies. Allergy. 2009;**64**:1109-1116.

[10] Hinchey EJ, Schaal PH, Richards MB. Treatment of perforated diverticular disease of the colon. Advances in surgery 1978;**12**:85-109.

[11] Neff CC, van Sonnenberg E. CT of diverticulitis. Diagnosis and treatment. Radiologic clinics of North America. 1989;**27**:743-752.

[12] Ambrosetti P, Becker C, Terrier F. Colonic diverticulitis: impact of imaging on surgical management—a prospective study of 542 patients. European radiology. 2002;**12**:1145-1149.

[13] Kaiser AM, Jiang JK, Lake JP, Ault G, Artinyan A, Gonzalez-Ruiz C, et al. The management of complicated diverticulitis and the role of computed tomography. The American journal of gastroenterology. 2005;**100**:910-917.

[14] Mora Lopez L, Serra Pla S, Serra-Aracil X, Ballesteros E, Navarro S. Application of a modified Neff classification to patients with uncomplicated diverticulitis. Colorectal disease. 2013;**15**:1442-1447.

[15] Sallinen VJ, Leppäniemi AK, Mentula PJ. Staging of acute diverticulitis based on clinical, radiologic, and physiologic parameters. The journal of trauma and acute care surgery. 2015;**78**:543-551.

[16] Sartelli M, Moore FA, Ansaloni L, Di Saverio S, Coccolini F, Griffiths EA, et al. A proposal for a CT driven classification of left colon acute diverticulitis. World journal of emergency surgery. 2015;**10**:3.

[17] Kechagias A, Rautio T, Kechagias G, Mäkelä J. The role of C-reactive protein in the prediction of the clinical severity of acute diverticulitis. The American surgeon. 2014;**80**:391-395.

[18] Van de Wall BJ, Draaisma WA, van der Kaaij RT, Consten EC, Wiezer MJ, Broeders IA. The value of inflammation markers and body temperature in acute diverticulitis. Colorectal disease. 2013;**15**:621-626.

[19] Mäkelä JT, Klintrup K, Takala H, Rautio T. The role of C-reactive protein in prediction of the severity of acute diverticulitis in an emergency unit. Scandinavian journal of gastroenterology. 2015;**50**:536-541.

[20] Laméris W, van Randen A, Bipat S, Bossuyt PM, Boermeester MA, Stoker J. Graded compression ultrasonography and computed tomography in acute colonic diverticulitis: meta- analysis of test accuracy. European radiology. 2008;**18**:2498-2511.

[21] Liljegren G, Chabok A, Wickbom M, Smedh K, Nilsson K. Acute colonic diverticulitis: a systematic review of diagnostic accuracy. Colorectal disease. 2007;**9**:480-488.

[22] Ambrosetti P, Jenny A, Becker C, Terrier TF, Morel P. Acute left colonic diverticulitis–compared performance of computed tomography and water-soluble contrast enema: prospective evaluation of 420 patients. Diseases of the colon and rectum. 2000;**43**: 1363-1367.

[23] Hwang SS, Cannom RR, Abbas MA, Etzioni D. Diverticulitis in transplant patients and patients on chronic corticosteroid therapy: a systematic review. Diseases of the colon and rectum. 2010;**53**:1699-1707.

[24] Dalla Valle R, Capocasale E, Mazzoni MP, Busi N, Benozzi L, Sivelli R, et al. Acute diverticulitis with colon perforation in renal transplantation. Transplantation proceedings. 2005;**37**:2507-2510.

[25] Qasabian RA, Meagher AP, Lee R, Dore GJ, Keogh A. Severe diverticulitis after heart, lung, and heart-lung transplantation. The Journal of heart and lung transplantation. 2004;**23**:845-849.

[26] Lederman ED, Conti DJ, Lempert N, Singh TP, Lee EC. Complicated diverticulitis following renal transplantation. Diseases of the colon and rectum. 1998;**41**:613-618.

[27] Bordeianou L, Hodin R. Controversies in the surgical management of sigmoid diverticulitis. Journal of gastrointestinal surgery. 2007;**11**:542-548.

[28] Biondo S, Trenti L, Elvira J, Golda T, Kreisler E. Outcomes of colonic diverticulitis according to the reason of immunosuppression. American journal of surgery. 2016;**21**:384-390.

[29] Sartelli M, Chichom-Mefire A, Labricciosa FM, Hardcastle T, Abu-Zidan FM, Adesunkanmi AK, et al. The management of intra-abdominal infections from a global perspective: 2017 WSES guidelines for management of intra-abdominal infections. World journal of emergency surgery. 2017;12:29. Erratum in: World journal of emergency surgery. 2017;**12**:36.

[30] Chabok A, Påhlman L, Hjern F, Haapaniemi S, Smedh K, AVOD Study Group. Randomized clinical trial of antibiotics in acute uncomplicated diverticulitis. The British journal of surgery. 2012;**99**:532-539.

[31] Sartelli M, Viale P, Catena F, Ansaloni L, Moore E, Malangoni M, et al. 2013 WSES guidelines for management of intra-abdominalinfections. World journal of emergency surgery. 2013;**8**:3.

[32] Ridgway PF, Latif A, Shabbir J, Ofriokuma F, Hurley MJ, Evoy D, et al. Randomized controlled trial of oral vs. intravenous therapy for the clinically diagnosed acute uncomplicated diverticulitis. Colorectal disease. 2009;**11**:941-946.

[33] Etzioni DA, Chiu VY, Cannom RR, Burchette RJ, Haigh PI, Abbas MA. Outpatient treatment of acute diverticulitis: rates and predictors of failure. Diseases of the colon and rectum. 2010;**53**:861-865.

[34] Jackson JD, Hammond T. Systematic review: outpatient management of acute uncomplicated diverticulitis. International journal of colorectal disease. 2014;**29**:775-781.

[35] Rodrìguez-Cerrillo M, Poza-Montoro A, Fernandez-Diaz E, Matesanz-David M, Inurrieta RA. Treatment of elderly patients with uncomplicated diverticulitis, even with comorbidity, at home. European journal of internal medicine. 2013;**24**:430-432.

[36] Biondo S, Golda T, Kreisler E, Espin E, Vallribera F, Oteiza F, et al. Outpatient versus hospitalization management for uncomplicated diverticulitis: a prospective, multicenter randomized clinical trial (DIVER trial). Annals of surgery. 2014;**259**:38-44.

[37] Andersen JC, Bundgaard L, Elbrønd H, Laurberg S, Walker LR, Støvring J, et al. Danish national guidelines for treatment of diverticular disease. Danish medical journal. 2012;**59**:C4453.

[38] Gregersen R, Mortensen LQ, Burcharth J, Pommergaard HC, Rosenberg J. Treatment of patients with acute colonic diverticulitis complicated by abscess formation: a systematic review. International journal of surgery. 2016;**35**:201-208.

[39] Ambrosetti P, Chautems R, Soravia C, Peiris-Waser N, Terrier F. Long-term outcome of mesocolic and pelvic diverticular abscesses of the left colon: a prospective study of 73 cases. Diseases of the colon and rectum. 2005;**48**:787-791.

[40] Brandt D, Gervaz P, Durmishi Y, Platon A, Morel P, Poletti PA. Percutaneous CT scan guided drainage versus antibiotherapy alone for Hinchey II diverticulitis: a case–control study. Diseases of the colon and rectum. 2006;**49**:1533-1538.

[41] Siewert B, Tye G, Kruskal J, Sosna J, Opelka F, Raptopoulos V, et al. Impact of CT-guided drainage in the treatment of diverticular abscesses: size matters. American journal of roentgenology. 2006;**186**:680-686.

[42] Singh B, May K, Coltart I, Moore NR, Cunningham C. The long-term results of percutaneous drainage of diverticular abscess. Annals of the Royal College of Surgeons of England. 2008;**90**:297-301.

[43] Kumar RR, Kim JT, Haukoos JS, Macias LH, Dixon MR, Stamos MJ, et al. Factors affecting the successful management of intra-abdominal abscesses with antibiotics and the need for percutaneous drainage. Diseases of the colon and rectum. 2006;**49**:183-189.

[44] Elagili F, Stocchi L, Ozuner G, Kiran RP. Antibiotics alone instead of percutaneous drainage as initial treatment of large diverticular abscess. Techniques in coloproctology. 2015;**19**:97-103.

[45] Feingold D, Steele SR, Lee S, Kaiser A, Boushey R, Buie WD, et al. Practice parameters for the treatment of sigmoid diverticulitis. Diseases of the colon and rectum. 2014;**57**:284-294.

[46] Dharmarajan S, Hunt SR, Birnbaum EH, Fleshman JW, Mutch MG. The efficacy of nonoperative management of acute

complicated diverticulitis. Diseases of the colon and rectum. 2011;**54**:663-671.

[47] Sallinen VJ, Mentula PJ, Leppäniemi AK. Nonoperative management of perforated diverticulitis with extraluminal air is safe and effective in selected patients. Diseases of the colon and rectum. 2014;**57**:875-881.

[48] Tsai HL, Hsieh JS, Yu FJ, Wu DC, Chen FM, Huang CJ, et al. Perforated colonic cancer presenting as intra-abdominal abscess. International journal of colorectal disease. 2007;**22**:15-19.

[49] Yeo ES, Ng KH, Eu KW. Perforated colorectal cancer: an important differential diagnosis in all presumed diverticular abscesses. Annals of the Academy of Medicine, Singapore. 2011;**40**:375-378.

[50] de Vries HS, Boerma D, Timmer R, van Ramshorst B, Dieleman LA, van Westreenen HL. Routine colonoscopy is not required in uncomplicated diverticulitis: a systematic review. Surgical endoscopy. 2014;**28**: 2039-2047.

[51] Rossi GL, Mentz R, Bertone S, Ojea Quintana G, Bilbao S, Im VM, et al. Laparoscopic peritoneal lavage for Hinchey III diverticulitis: is it as effective as it is applicable? Diseases of the colon and rectum. 2014;**57**:1384-1390.

[52] Swank HA, Mulder IM, Hoofwijk AG, Nienhuijs SW, Lange JF, Bemelman WA. Dutch diverticular disease collaborative study G. early experience with laparoscopic lavage for perforated diverticulitis. The British journal of surgery. 2013;**100**:704-710.

[53] Schultz JK, Yaqub S, Wallon C, Blecic L, Forsmo HM, Folkesson J, et al. Laparoscopic lavage vs. primary resection for acute perforated diverticulitis: the SCANDIV randomized clinical trial. JAMA. 2015;**314**:1364-1375.

[54] Vennix S, Musters GD, Mulder IM, Swank HA, Consten EC, Belgers EH, et al. Laparoscopic peritoneal lavage or sigmoidectomy for perforated diverticulitis with purulent peritonitis: a multicentre, parallel-group, randomized, open-label trial. Lancet. 2015;**386**(10000):1269-1277.

[55] McCafferty MH, Roth L, Jorden J. Current management of diverticulitis. The American surgeon. 2008;**74**:1041-1049.

[56] Fleming FJ, Gillen P. Reversal of Hartmann's procedure following acute diverticulitis: is timing everything? International journal of colorectal disease. 2009;**24**:1219-1225.

[57] Lee JM, Bai P, Chang J, El Hechi M, Kongkaewpaisan N, Bonde A, et al. Hartmann's procedure vs. primary anastomosis with diverting loop ileostomy for acute diverticulitis: nationwide analysis of 2,729 emergency surgery patients. Journal of the American College of Surgeons. 2019;**229**:48-55.

[58] Oberkofler CE, Rickenbacher A, Raptis DA, Lehmann K, Villiger P, Buchli C, et al. A multicenter randomized clinical trial of primary anastomosis or Hartmann's procedure for perforated left colonic diverticulitis with purulent or fecal peritonitis. Annals of surgery. 2012;**256**:819-826.

[59] Lambrichts DPV, Vennix S, Musters GD, Mulder IM, Swank HA, Hoofwijk AGM, et al. Hartmann's procedure versus sigmoidectomy with primary anastomosis for perforated diverticulitis with purulent or fecal peritonitis (LADIES): a multicentre, parallel-group, randomized, open-label, superiority trial. The lancet. Gastroenterology & hepatology. 2019;**4**:599-610.

[60] Halim H, Askari A, Nunn R, Hollingshead J. Primary resection anastomosis versus Hartmann's procedure in Hinchey III and IV diverticulitis. World journal of emergency surgery. 2019;**14**:32.

[61] Vennix S, Boersema GS, Buskens CJ, Menon AG, Tanis PJ, Lange JF, et al. Emergency laparoscopic sigmoidectomy for perforated diverticulitis with generalized peritonitis: a systematic review. Digestive surgery. 2016; **33**:1-7.

[62] Kafka-Ritsch R, Birkfellner F, Perathoner A, Raab H, Nehoda H, Pratschke J, et al. Damage control surgery with abdominal vacuum and delayed bowel reconstruction in patients with perforated diverticulitis Hinchey III/IV. Journal of gastrointestinal surgery 2012;**16**:1915-1922.

[63] Ordóñez CA, Sánchez AI, Pineda JA, Badiel M, Mesa R, Cardona U, et al. Deferred primary anastomosis versus diversion in patients with severe secondary peritonitis managed with staged laparotomies. World journal of emergency surgery. 2010;**34**:169-176.

[64] Sartelli M, Catena F, Abu-Zidan FM, Ansaloni L, Biffl WL, Boermeester MA, et al. Management of intra-abdominal infections: recommendations by the WSES 2016 consensus conference. World journal of emergency surgery. 2017;**12**:22.

[65] Kirkpatrick AW, Coccolini F, Ansaloni L, Roberts DJ, Tolonen M, McKee JL, et al. Closed or open after laparotomy (COOL) after source control for severe complicated intra-abdominal sepsis investigators. Closed or open after source control laparotomy for severe complicated intra-abdominal sepsis (the COOL trial): study protocol for a randomized controlled trial. World journal of emergency surgery. 2018;**13**:26.

[66] Rafferty J, Shellito P, Hyman NH, Buie WD. Standards Committee of the American Society of colon and Rectal surgeons. Practice parameters for sigmoid diverticulitis. Diseases of the colon and rectum. 2006;**49**:939-944.

[67] Hall JF, Roberts PL, Ricciardi R, Read T, Scheirey C, Wald C, et al. Long-term follow-up after an initial episode of diverticulitis: what are the predictors of recurrence? Diseases of the colon and rectum. 2011;**54**: 283-288.

[68] El-Sayed C, Radley S, Mytton J, Evison F, Ward ST. Risk of recurrent disease and surgery following an admission for acute diverticulitis. Diseases of the colon and rectum. 2018;**61**:382-389.

[69] van de Wall BJM, Stam MAW, Draaisma WA, Stellato R, Bemelman WA, Boermeester MA, et al. Surgery versus conservative management for recurrent and ongoing left-sided diverticulitis (DIRECT trial): an open-label, multicentre, randomized controlled trial. The lancet. Gastroenterology & hepatology. 2017;**2**:13-22.

[70] Klarenbeek BR, Samuels M, van der Wal MA, van der Peet DL, Meijerink WJ, Cuesta MA. Indications for elective sigmoid resection in diverticular disease. Annals of surgery. 2010;**251**:670-674.

[71] Halpenny DF, McNeil G, Snow A, Geoghegan T, Torreggiani WC. Prospective evaluation of the value of magnetic resonance imaging in suspected acute sigmoid diverticulitis. Diseases of the colon and rectum. 2009;**52**:1030-1031.

[72] Sawyer RG, Claridge JA, Nathens AB, Rotstein OD, Duane TM, Evans HL, et al. Trial of short-course antimicrobial therapy for intraabdominal infection. The New

England journal of medicine. 2015;**372**:1996-2005.

[73] Chiu TC, Chou YH, Tiu CM, Chiou HJ, Wang HK, Lai YC, et al. Right-sided colonic diverticulitis: clinical features, sonographic appearances, and management. Journal of medical ultrasound. 2017;**25**:33-39.

[74] Ha GW, Lee MR, Kim JH. Efficacy of conservative management in patients with right colonic diverticulitis. Australian and New Zealand journal of surgery. 2017;**87**:467-470.

[75] Kim SH, Byun CG, Cha JW, Choi SH, Kho YT, Seo DY. Comparative study of the clinical features and treatment for right and left colonic diverticulitis. Journal of the Korean Society of Coloproctology. 2010;**26**:407-412.

[76] Kim JY, Park SG, Kang HJ, Lim YA, Pak KH, Yoo T, et al. Prospective randomized clinical trial of uncomplicated right-sided colonic diverticulitis: antibiotics versus no antibiotics. International journal of colorectal disease. 2019;**34**:1413-1420.

[77] Destek S, Gül VO. Effectiveness of conservative approach in right colon diverticulitis. Turkish journal of trauma & emergency surgery. 2019;**25**:396-402.

[78] Chung BH, Ha GW, Lee MR, Kim JH. Management of colonic diverticulitis tailored to location and severity: comparison of the right and the left colon. Annals of coloproctology. 2016;**32**:228-233.

[79] Mesina C, Dumitrescu TV, Obleaga CV, Ciobanu D, Ischemic colitis problems of diagnosis and treatment, Archive of Clinical and Experimental Surgery. 2018;**7**:59-64.

[80] Meşină C, Vasile I, Paşalega M, Calotă F, Vîlcea D. Ischemia acută mezenterică, Chirurgia, 2008, **103**(4): 378-388.

[81] Vasile I, Meşină C, Paşalega M, Calotă F, Vîlcea ID, Ischemie acută mezenterică non-ocluzivă, Chirurgia, 2008, **103**(3):337-343.

Chapter 4

Inflammatory Complication of Diverticular Disease

Luciano Dias de Oliveira Reis,
Marcos Ricardo da Silva Rodrigues,
Celso Augusto Milani Cardoso Filho,
Cassiana Franco Dias dos Reis and Alex Antonio de Paula Costa

Abstract

Diverticular disease is the most common morphological abnormality of the colon. It is increasing in prevalence proportionally to progressive aging and modern alimentary diet. The majority of the diverticular disease affects the sigmoid colon and the segmental inflammatory process can have different outcomes, from self-limited, low-grade inflammation to severe cases evolving to complications such as abscess, fistulas to different organs, free perforation and peritonitis, sepsis, intestinal obstruction, and hemorrhage. In this chapter, we will focus on a few of these complications—focal low-grade inflammation, intra-abdominal abscess, and fistulas.

Keywords: diverticular disease, diverticulitis, complicated diverticulitis, intra-abdominal abscess, sigmoid fistulas

1. Introduction

The incidence of diverticular disease (DD) has been rising in the last years, affecting 50–60% of people at the age of 60 [1, 2]. Only 20% of the patients with DD will develop symptoms, without acute inflammatory signs. Even so, the majority of them will be treated conservatively with success, but in some cases, complications such as abscess, obstruction, hemorrhage, perforation, and fistula will arise [3–5].

The majority of the diverticular disease affects the sigmoid colon. Its inflammatory process can have different outcomes, from self-limited, low-grade inflammation to severe cases evolving to abscess or perforation of the colonic wall. The perforation may have different presentations—free perforations when the colon communicates with the peritoneal cavity or can be walled off by the omentum or surrounding viscera.

Free perforation of the colon results in peritonitis and demands urgent surgical treatment.

Low-grade inflammation may cause tiny breaches and involve adjacent peritoneum, viscera, and mesentery fat, resulting in acute inflammatory reactions. Adhesion of surrounding structures will result in an inflammatory mass. Usually, it will result in walled-off infection and abscesses, which may heal with medical treatment. Sometimes, the abscess may need to be drained surgically or aided by the radiological guide.

This inflammatory process may erode to the adhered organ and cause an internal fistula, notably the urinary bladder, but also to the small bowel, uterus, vagina or may erode through the abdominal wall resulting in an external fistula.

Also, the inflammatory reaction resulted from acute diverticulitis may result in intestinal obstruction and bleeding but these issues will be in another chapter.

2. Abscess

2.1 Abscess following acute diverticulitis

In a small number of patients with acute diverticulitis, the complication will appear. The abscess is one of the potentially hazardous complications. It may be a small phlegmon, pericolic, pelvic, or even distant. The management can be nonoperatively or surgical. Little has changed in the last decades except for the important improvement in decision-making based on the recent progress of radiological images. Clinical observation and daily examination are still the most important steps.

The majority of diverticular disease affects the sigmoid colon and the segmental inflammatory process can have different outcomes, from self-limited, low-grade inflammation to severe cases evolving to the abscess.

The success of medical management for diverticular disease depends on the patient's presentation and degree of response to treatment. The patient's presentation can be grouped into categories based on the Hinchey classification [6].

Clinical presentation, physical examination, and diagnostics studies help to group patients.

Patients with complicated diverticulitis present with different forms, from mild to severe cases. They may present as phlegmon, pericolic or distant abscesses, and peritonitis as shown in **Table 1**.

Mild disease can often be managed with diet, anti-inflammatory, antibiotics, and close observation on an outpatient basis (Hinchey 0 and Ia) but more severe cases should be hospitalized. The more severe cases are classified as Hinchey Ib and II.

Daily physical examination, laboratory blood checks, and CT scan help to follow the progression of the disease. The two most common signs of diverticulitis on CT scan are bowel wall thickening and fat stranding [7]. CT scan is so important that helps to links the clinical presentation to the modified Hinchey classification [6, 8].

Stage	Description
Modified Hinchey classification	
0	Mild clinical diverticulitis
Ia	Confined pericolic inflammation or phlegmon
Ib	Confined pericolic abscess
II	Pelvic, distant intra-abdominal or retroperitoneal abscess
III	Generalized purulent peritonitis
IV	Generalized fecal peritonitis

Table 1.
Modified Hinchey classification.

Patients Hinchey 0 and IB may be treated conservatively, even on an outpatient basis but require daily follow-up. Small perforation with pneumoperitoneum identified on CT scan in a patient with minimal symptoms has been treated conservatively on an outpatient basis. Extraluminal air alone is not an indication for emergency surgery but close monitoring is mandatory to detect treatment failure early [9].

Patients with pneumoperitoneum with virtually no symptoms may be treated conservatively on an outpatient basis (**Figure 1**). Even patients with pneumoperitoneum far away from the diverticular site may be treated conservatively (**Figure 2**).

In this case, the patient was kept in hospital for 72 hours and he was sent home asymptomatic. Patients in stages Ib and II can be managed with the combination of antibiotics, bowel rest, analgesics, and intravenous fluids. As they improve the antibiotics, fluid replacement may be offered by mouth. There are a number of papers comparing the results of many different antibiotics [7].

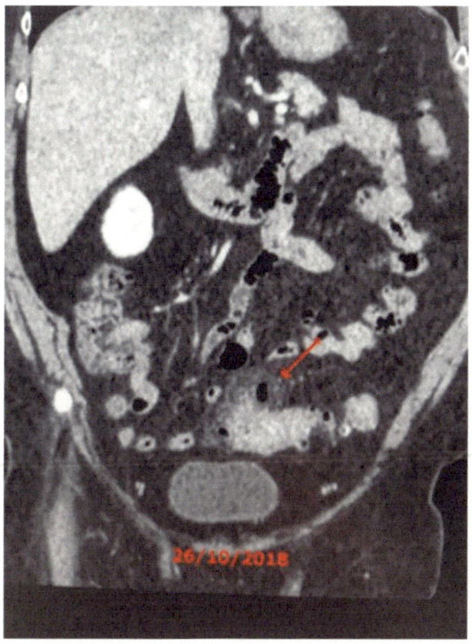

Figure 1.
Pneumoperitoneum in oligosymptomatic patient (Hinchey I).

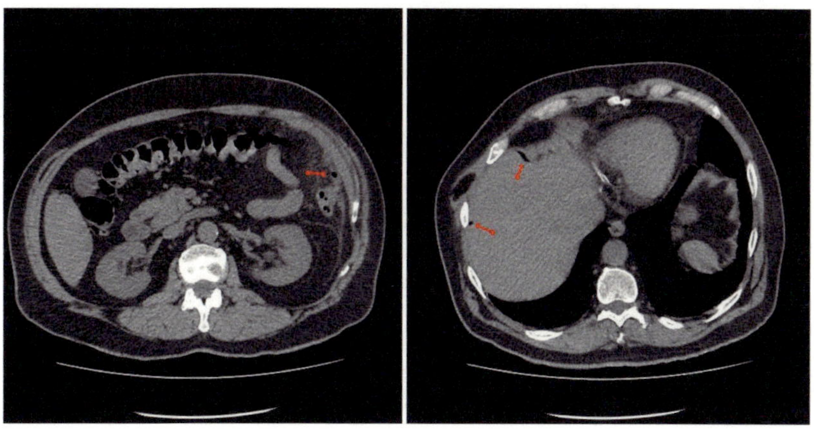

Figure 2.
Several small spots of pneumoperitoneum.

For an outpatient oral regimen, a fluoroquinolone as levofloxacin or ciprofloxacin associated with metronidazole or clindamycin is a two-drug combination. For patient on intravenous regimen, ciprofloxacin or third-generation cephalosporin is associated with metronidazole or clindamycin.

The patients should be switched from IV to oral therapy when they accept oral medicines and diet. The turning point of the transition from IV to oral medication and feeding is based on clinical improvement and it is linked to the doctor's feelings. Serial radiological studies also give important support to the physician.

According to the ASRS, Practice Parameters for sigmoid diverticulitis "radiological guided percutaneous drainage is usually the most appropriate treatment for patients with large diverticular abscess." They recommend hospitalization and IV antibiotics for these patients. If the abscess is smaller than 2 cm in diameter, it may resolve with antibiotics alone, whereas a larger abscess should be percutaneously drained [7, 10].

Some of these patients will not respond favorably to medical treatment and will develop a complication from their abscesses. How to treat pos diverticulitis abscess is debatable. This condition also can be treated clinically associated or not with percutaneous drainage. If clinical treatment fails, we must consider surgical drainage, by laparoscopy or laparotomy.

The location and size of the abscess are of importance. Siewart et al. published an interesting retrospective study comparing the outcome of abscess related to its size. They had a successful treatment in all 22 patients who were treated with antibiotics and clinical support for abscesses up to 3 cm in size [11]. Ambrosetti et al. published a prospective study and found that pelvic abscesses were more likely to require surgery if they were pelvic than mesocolic. Their recommendations were to drain all pelvic abscesses and mesocolic abscesses that were more than 5 cm in size or if no improvement after initial antibiotics [12].

Figure 3 refer to an obese patient with a large intra-abdominal abscess treated by percutaneous drainage of 200 ml of pus. The patient improved and was at the latter date submitted to sigmoid colectomy with good results.

An excellent recent systematic review (Fowler, 2021) stated the definition for the failure of nonoperative management, as a need for emergency or urgent surgery during the index admission. Other criteria were persistent or enlarging of

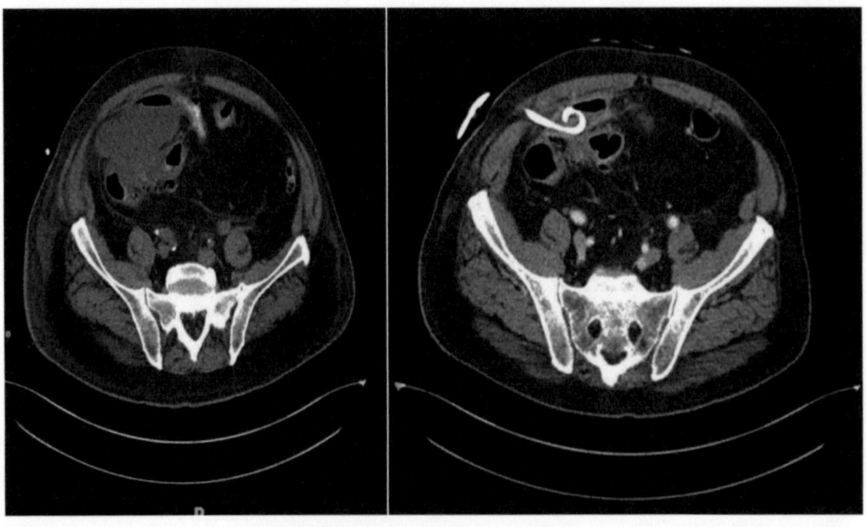

Figure 3.
Large abscess drained percutaneously under radiological guidance.

the abscess, persistent or worsening sepsis, development of complications, such as peritonitis, ileus, fistula, persistent percutaneous drainage from the percutaneous puncture site. The same study showed that the failure rate of nonoperative management, which included 38 studies (n = 2598), was 16.4%. In the same study, the failure rate for percutaneous drainage was 17% for pericolic and 44% for pelvic abscess [13].

After initial successful nonoperative management of diverticular abscess, expectant management with nonoperative intent is a safe long-term option with low rates of surgery [14].

When conservative treatment fails, surgery is indicated.

Sometimes, the abscess is not feasible to conservative treatment due to its inaccessibility. It may not be punctured safely. Occasionally, the abscess is intramesenteric and cannot be rained percutaneously and a sigmoid resection is mandatory (**Figures 4** and **5**).

One of the criteria for failure is the recurrence of diverticulitis. The number of recurrent episodes as criteria for elective surgery is still controverted [7]. Elective operation achieves the best results. Emergency surgical procedure has a higher morbidity and mortality rate and is related to Hinchey's classification. Surgical techniques had not changed for years, and range from surgical drainage of the abscess, associated with lavage of the abdominal cavity by laparotomy or recently *via* laparoscopy and resection of the diseased colon with primary anastomosis associated or not with the protective stoma or Hartmann's procedure that is the resection of the diseased colon with the closure of distal bowel and proximal colostomy.

These operations will be discussed later in this book.

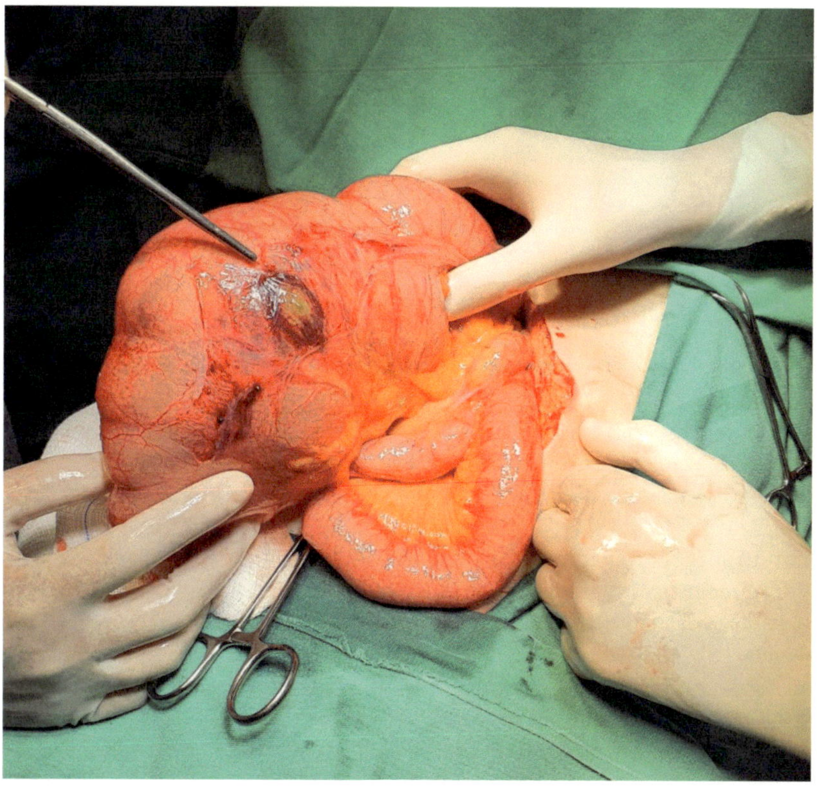

Figure 4.
Large mesocolic abscess.

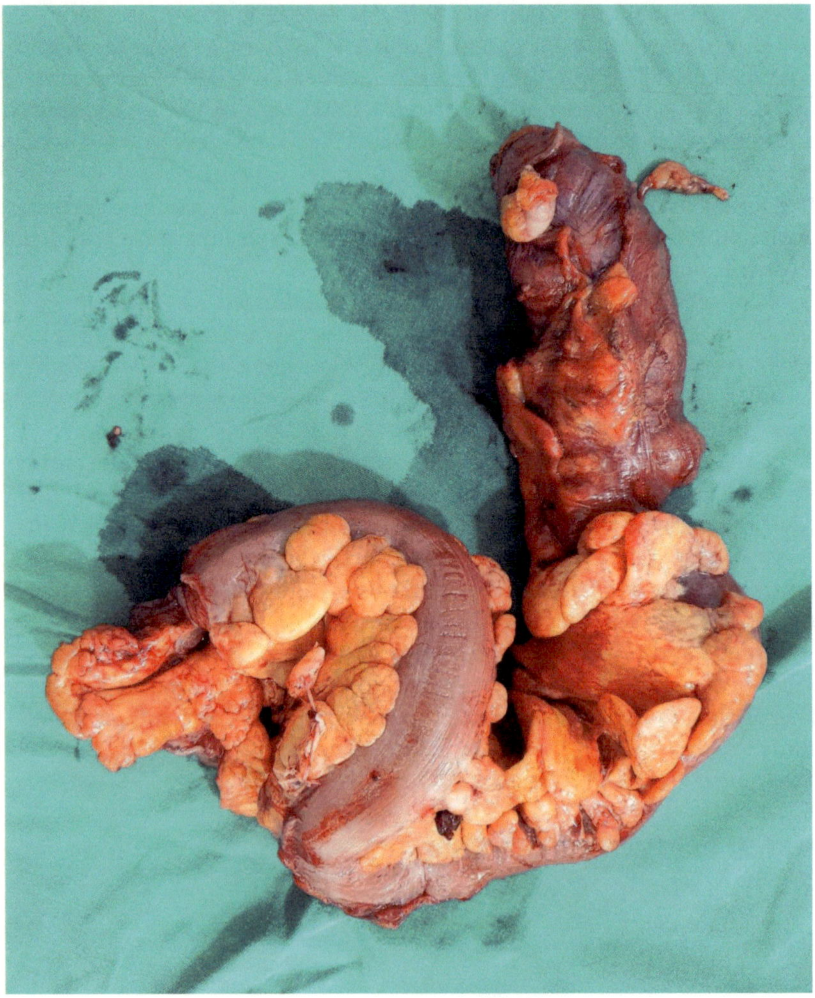

Figure 5.
Surgical removed left colon with chronic diverticulitis, with mesocolic abscess.

3. Fistulas

Chronically, the local inflammatory process can give rise to fistulas from the sigmoid to many adjacent organs. The most common etiology for colovesical fistula is a diverticular disease (40–80%) but CVF can also be found in cancer (19%), Crohn's disease, radiotherapy, or iatrogenesis [15].

Among patients with diverticulitis, only a few will develop complications as fistula [2, 3, 16, 17].

Open surgery management has been the standard treatment for these fistulas. More recently, laparoscopic surgery has shown to be an alternative and less invasive approach even though it is described to have high conversion rates up to 46.9% [2]. The American Society of Colon and Rectal Surgeons Practice Parameters recommends the laparoscopic approach when the expertise is available [5, 15].

Symptoms of the fistula depend on the organs involved. The bladder is the most common site from fistulas originating from sigmoid diverticulitis (65–69%) but is followed by vagina (25%), intestine (6%), skin (6%) [2, 6, 18], and very rarely to the appendix, tubes, and uterus.

3.1 Sigmoidvesical fistula

The pathogenesis is related to inflammation leading to perforation of the diverticulum and overt communication to a previously organ. When the adherence is to the bladder, it may erode through the bladder's wall resulting in a sigmoid vesical fistula.

Colovesical fistula secondary to diverticulitis occurs in up to 5% of patients with complicated diverticulitis and its incidence is rising [15, 19].

Diagnosis is often based on pathognomonic signs—fecaluria, pneumaturia, and recurrent urinary infection [4, 19, 20] in a patient with a history of symptomatic diverticular disease.

Sigmoidovesical fistula is more common in elder males and in women who have been submitted to hysterectomy [5]. These observations support the theory that the body and fundus of the uterus may act as a protective barrier [15, 21]. In our recently published cases, all six patients were males [22]. Between 1999 and 2019, we had six patients with sigmoidovesical fistula. A summary of these patients is shown in **Table 2**.

All the reported patients were male. All patients treated under elective conditions (n = 3) were given primary colonic resection and anastomosis of the colon and presented uneventful recovery. The last treated patient was the only one submitted to the laparoscopic approach. In this case, intense fibrosis between the bladder and colon wall was found. The urinary bladder fistula orifice was not identified, and the bladder was not sutured. The urinary catheter was left *in situ* for 2 weeks. In all five laparotomic patients, the bladder was sutured.

Ultrasound, cystoscopy, and CT are used to confirm the diagnosis, but CT is the most accurate, showing up to 90% of sensibility, and considered the gold standard for detection of colovesical fistula [5, 23, 24]. MRI is highly sensitive but it is expensive and less accessible [15, 25]. In the last few years, CT became available in most places and was used in our recent cases (**Figure 6**).

Surgery is the method of choice for sigmoidovesical fistula. Only the unfit patient should be treated conservatively [26]. Surgery consists of removing the diseased segment of the colon, as well as the fistula, with the primary suture of the bladder defect, when identified, to prevent recurrence (**Figure 7**) [23].

Cases	Age	Symptoms	Procedures	Complications
1	70	Urinary sepsis, pneumaturia, abdominal pain, emphysema	Hartmann	X
2	65	Dysuria, pneumaturia, abdominal pain, fever	Hartmann colorectal anastomosis after 3 months	X
3	63	Recurrent crises of diverticulitis. Pneumaturia	Resection and anastomosis	X
4	38	Recurrent urinary infection, dysuria, pneumaturia, and abdominal pain	Resection and anastomosis	X
5	39	Pneumaturia, palpable mass in the hypogastrium	Hartmann colorectal anastomosis after 7 months	Partial wound dehiscence
6	56	Left lower abdominal pain, fever, pneumaturia, and foul urine	Laparoscopic resection and anastomosis	X

Table 2.
Authors' experience with sigmoidovesical fistula.

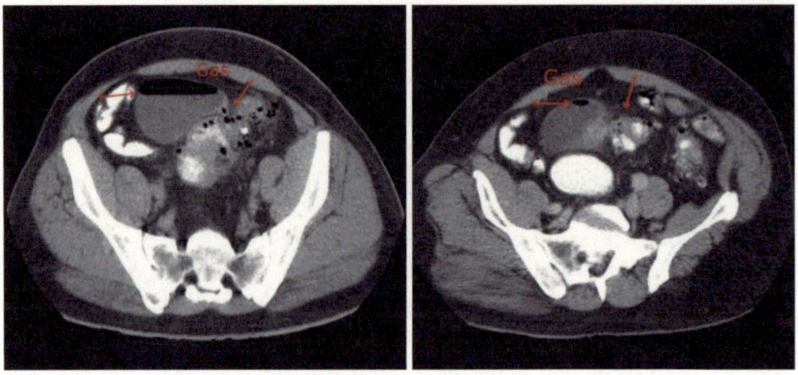

Figure 6.
Note air inside de bladder and signs of diverticulitis.

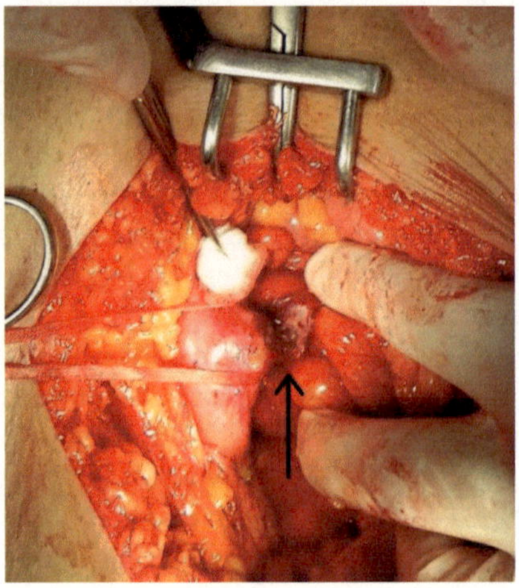

Figure 7.
Fistula tract from the sigmoid colon to the bladder.

In high-risk cases, it may not be safe to proceed to the primary anastomosis, and Hartmann's procedure is a good option [5, 23, 27]. This procedure can be performed *via* laparotomy and laparoscopy, and there are a few reports on robotic [2, 18].

The laparoscopic approach has been progressively performed [2, 6, 25]. Recent studies of laparoscopic management of complicated diverticulitis have demonstrated that under experienced hands, operation time and conversion rates are acceptable, and morbidity and mortality rates are compared with open surgery [1–3, 17, 25, 26]. Currently, the American Society of Colon and Rectal Surgeons Practice Parameters recommends a laparoscopic approach for elective colectomies when expertise is available [2, 5].

Martinolich et al. reported in 2018, the outcome of 111 patients with diverticula fistulas submitted to minimally invasive sigmoid colectomy with primary anastomosis [2]. Five patients were unfit for the method and excluded from the study. The remaining 106 underwent sigmoid colectomy with primary anastomosis with a conversion rate of 34.7%. Four of these patients had a robotic approach without conversion. They concluded that laparoscopic sigmoid colectomy for CVF is safe, with results similar to open sigmoid resection. These results are supported by other reports [1, 5].

A 14-year surgery group experience treating CVF also demonstrated similar results when open and laparoscopic approaches were compared [17]. Recent reports compared robotic to laparoscopic approaches in colectomies and also found similar results. The only significant differences were prolonged operative time and higher costs in the robotic group [18, 20, 28].

A controversial issue is the management of the bladder site of the fistula. We performed the primary suture of the bladder in all of our open cases. Some authors claim that if the fistula orifice of the bladder wall is not easily found, it may be let without suture [23, 29]. Others claim that intraoperative instillation of methylene blue may be used to limit unnecessary bladder repair [6, 29]. The suture of the bladder is more frequently described in open approaches [17] possibly because it is less technically demanding under open access and also more common when the surgery is performed by general surgeons compared to urologists [29].

3.2 Sigmoidovaginal fistula

This complication is similar to a colovesical fistula. The inflammatory diverticular process may transform into an abscess and erode to the adhered vagina.

Sigmoidovaginal fistula is a relatively modern disease, being largely absent from medical literature until half of the last century [30]. It is related to the more common practice of hysterectomy in recent years. Still, it remains relatively rare.

The majority of patients are diagnosed by a gynecologist.

A triad for diagmosis of sigmoidvaginal fistula are as follows: 1. Patient reports stool and / or flatus per vagina or persistent foul-smelling vaginal discharge and vaginitis resistant to local medival treatment; 2. Previous hysterectomy; 3. History of diverticulosis or diverticulitis [31, 32].

The colovaginal fistula begins with inflammation, which typically affecting a loop of the sigmoid colon in the left side of the female pelvis. The inflamed sigmoid colon becomes adherent to the vaginal apex, either due to the diverticular inflammation or from previous adhesive disease. Then, a small abscess can form and drain through the convenient exit site of the vagina, leading to fistula formation. The sequence of events is similar to other fistulas arising from the diseased sigmoid colon.

It is interesting that among sigmoid fistulas complicating diverticulitis, colovesical and coloenteric fistulas are more common. Occasionally, internal fistulas complicating diverticulitis may open into the appendix, uterus, or tubes [33, 34].

Sigmoid vaginal fistulas are rare and usually affect patients submitted to hysterectomy. In a group of 19 patients, the interval between patients' hysterectomy and presentation for fistulas was 19 years, with a range of 1–39 years [31]. In this study, 89.5% of patients reported stool and 36.8% flatus per vagina.

Females have the interposition of the uterus between the sigmoid colon and the bladder and it occupies the *cull de sac*, pushing the sigmoid away from the vagina. **Figure 8** are from patients submitted to hysterectomy 35 years previously showing pelvic abscess, inflamed sigmoid, and air in the vagina. In Brazil, Safatle reported three cases, all of them in females submitted to hysterectomies and the fistulous tract was found in the proximal vagina [35].

The most common etiology for sigmoidovaginal fistula is a diverticular disease (40–80%) but it may also be found in cancer, Crohn's disease, radiotherapy, or iatrogenesis [15].

Gynecological examination is mandatory. The vaginal orifice of the colovaginal fistula will be visualized in 78.9% of 19 patients in a recent report [31]. Surgical scars of laparotomy or laparoscopy for hysterectomy are commonly found. These

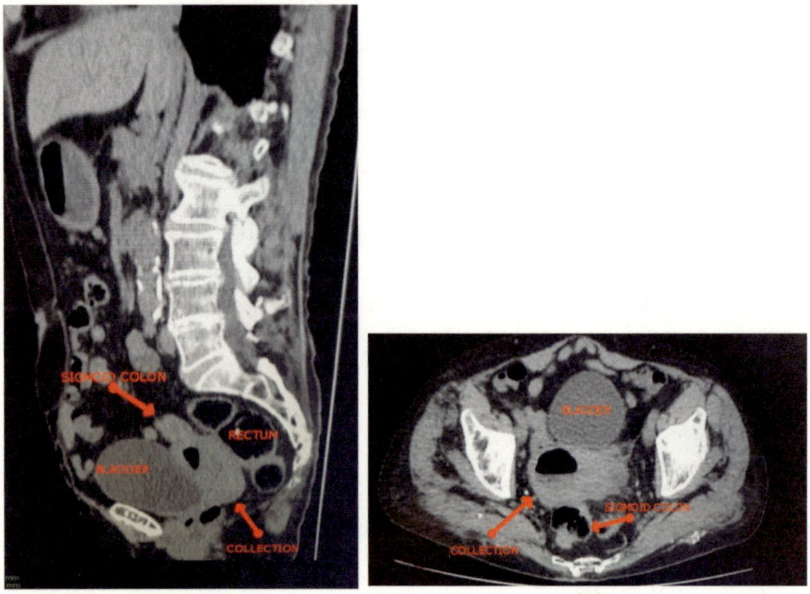

(a) (b)

Figure 8.
Pelvic abscess with sigmoidovaginal fistula.

observations support the theory that the body and fundus of the uterus may act as a protective barrier [15, 23, 30]. Conventional fluoroscopic evaluation of the vagina, or vaginography, involves the insertion of a catheter into the vagina, with a balloon inflated to create necessary filling pressure and distention. Water-soluble contrast material should be used and barium should be avoided [36].

CT is the gold-standard method that is used to confirm the diagnosis. It is accurate, showing up to 90% of sensibility, and is considered the gold standard for the detection of sigmoid fistulas [5, 23, 26]. MRI is highly sensitive but it is expensive and less accessible [15, 25]. In the last few years, CT scan became available in most places. MRI is an excellent method to identify the fistula's tract mainly if it affects the rectum and anal sphincter [36].

Surgery is the method of choice for sigmoidovaginal fistula [31]. Only patients at high risk of perioperative morbidity and mortality should be treated conservatively [26]. Surgery consists of removing the diseased segment of the colon, as well as the fistula, with primary suture of the vaginal defect, when identified, to prevent recurrence [23]. Omentum, peritoneum, or epiploic fat are frequently used to avoid recurrence but Fallopian salpinges have been used as well [31, 37].

In high-risk cases or locally complicated cases, it may not be safe to proceed to the primary anastomosis, and Hartmann's procedure is a good option [5, 23, 27]. This procedure can be performed *via* laparotomy, laparoscopy, or potentially through robotic surgery [2, 18].

A laparoscopic approach has been increasingly favored [2, 6, 15] as mentioned before [2]. The authors concluded that laparoscopic sigmoid colectomy for sigmoid fistula is safe, with results similar to open sigmoid resection. Recent reports compared robotic versus laparoscopic approach in colectomies and also found similar results. The only significant differences were prolonged operative time and higher costs in the robotic group [18, 20]. These reports are on larger groups of patients with sigmoidovesical fistulas, but the surgical approach applies to sigmoidovaginal fistulas. We mentioned them because since fistula to the bladder is more common than to vagina, the number of patients of the former groups is statistically significant.

Occasionally, the fistula involves various organs, such as the colon, bladder, and vagina, and needs a multidisciplinary approach [38].

A controversial issue is the management of the vaginal site of the fistula. Some authors claim that if the fistula orifice of the vagina or bladder may not be easily found, it may be let without suture [23, 29, 32]. The success rate of primary repair in healthy patients is high, approaching 95% [32].

Dessole reported interposition of Fallopian salpinges in the treatment of sigmoidovaginal fistula, secondary to vaginal hysterectomy with failure of previous repair [37].

The suture of the vagina is more frequently described in open approaches [17] possibly because it is less technically demanding under open access and also more common when the surgical procedure is performed by general surgeons [18]. Several studies have shown that long-term success seems independent of vaginal repair [31, 39, 40].

Sigmoidovaginal fistula is an unpleasant complication of diverticulitis and is increasingly common due to an aging population, it is an important presentation of which to be aware. These patients present with a triad—discharge of stool, flatus or malodorous vaginal secretion, diverticulitis, and history of hysterectomy. Surgical resection of the diseased sigmoid colon and primary anastomosis without repair of the vaginal defect is the ideal treatment. Close collaboration between gynecologists and colorectal surgeons promotes optimal care and management of this distressing condition.

3.3 Other sigmoid fistulas

Fistulas may occur from the diseased sigmoid to the Fallopian tubes, uterus, appendix, cecum, rectum, small intestine. Some coloenteric fistulas may be asymptomatic if the fistula is hermetically blocked, but they may also cause intestinal obstruction when an unsuspected fistula will be found.

Occasionally, the fistula will be driven to the skin, initially simulating a subcutaneous abscess eventually draining spontaneously, like the "empyema necessitatis," transforming into a sigmoid cutaneous fistula (**Figure 9**). A temporary sigmoidocutaneous fistula may arise as a consequence of percutaneous drainage of an abscess. Both will require a definitive surgical procedure.

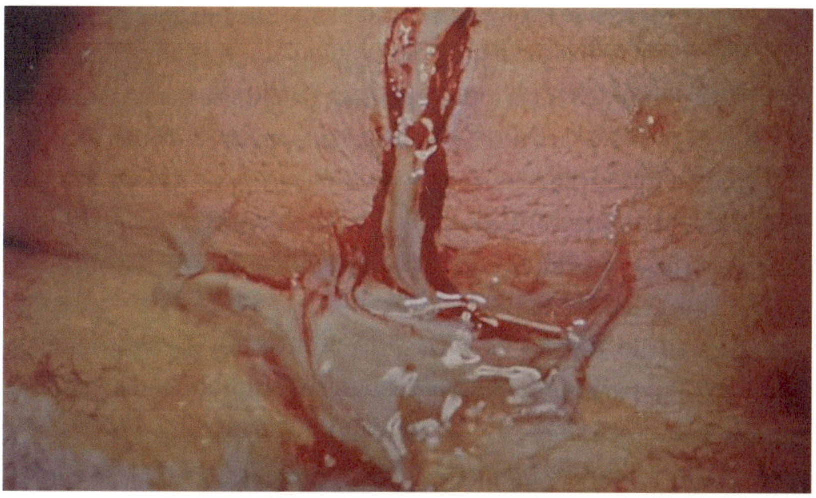

Figure 9.
Sigmoidocutaneos fistula following diverticulitis and abscess (courtesy of Enio C. Oliveira).

Fistulas to blood vessel are extremely rare but recently have been increasingly reported since some of them are secondary to vascular procedures [41]. Diverticulitis has been reported as a cause for primary sigmoidovascular fistulas associated or not with aortic aneurysms [41, 42]. The main symptom is massive bleeding, associated with vascular or diverticular symptoms. Bleeding may cause hypotension and generally is associated with sepsis due to direct contact of bowel content to the circulation. It is a dreadful complication of diverticulitis and carries a very high mortality rate. The treatment is bowel resection with or without colostomy and aortic graft replacement.

4. Conclusion

Diverticular disease may be complicated by acute inflammation, named diverticulitis. The majority of episodes of diverticulitis are mild and will be treated conservatively. Some cases will cause severe symptoms and are related to complications such as phlegmon, abscess, and fistulas. Phlegmon and abscesses may be treated conservatively but they require close observation. If it does not improve, they demand surgery. Fistulas are the undesirable complication of diverticulitis and their symptoms are directly related to the organ involved. Surgical treatment nearly always will be necessary and it includes sigmoid resection.

Author details

Luciano Dias de Oliveira Reis[1,2,3,4]*, Marcos Ricardo da Silva Rodrigues[2,5], Celso Augusto Milani Cardoso Filho[1,2,6], Cassiana Franco Dias dos Reis[4,7] and Alex Antonio de Paula Costa[4]

1 Brazilian College of Surgeons, Rio de Janeiro, Brazil

2 Brazilian Society of Colo-Proctology, Rio de Janeiro, Brazil

3 Brazilian Society of Digestive Endoscopy, Rio de Janeiro, Brazil

4 Hospital Nossa Senhora da Saúde, Santo Antônio da Platina, Paraná, Brazil

5 Department of Surgery, State University of Ponta Grossa, Paraná, Brazil

6 Hospital Sirio Libanes, São Paulo, Brazil

7 Coordinator of Department of Surgery, Hospital Nossa Senhora da Saúde, Santo Antônio da Platina, Paraná, Brazil

*Address all correspondence to: reisluciano@uol.com.br

References

[1] Bhakta A, Tafen M, Glotzer O, Canete J, Chismark AD, Valerian BT, et al. Laparoscopic sigmoid colectomy for complicated diverticulitis is safe: Review of 576 consecutive colectomies. Surgical Endoscopy. Apr 2016;**30**(4):1629-34

[2] Martinolich J, Croasdale DR, Bhakta AS, Ata A, Chismark AD, Valerian BT, et al. Laparoscopic surgery for diverticular fistulas: Outcomes of 111 consecutive cases at a single institution. Journal of Gastrointestinal Surgery. May 2019;**23**(5):1015-21

[3] Cirocchi R, Cochetti G, Randolph J, Listorti C, Castellani E, Renzi C, et al. Laparoscopic treatment of C due to complicated colonic diverticular disease: A systematic review. Techniques in Coloproctology. 2014;**18**(10):873-85

[4] Cochetti G, Del Zingaro M, Boni A, Cocca D, Panciarola M, Tiezzi A, et al. Colovesical fistula: Review on conservative management, surgical techiniques and minimaly invasive approaches. Il Giornale di Chirurgia. 2018;**39**(4):195-207

[5] Feingold D, Steele RS, Lee S, Kaiser A, Boushey R, Donald Buie W, et al. Practice parameters for the treatment of sigmoid diverticulitis. Diseases of the Colon and Rectum. 2014;**57**:284-294

[6] Hinchey EJ, Schaal PG, Richards GK. Treatment of perforated diverticular disease of the colon. Advances in Surgery. 1978;**12**:85-109

[7] Beckham H, Whitlow CB. The medical and nonoperative treatment of diverticulitis. Clinics in Colon and Rectal Surgery. Aug 2009;**22**(3):156-60. doi:10.1055/s-0029-1236159

[8] Keiser AM, Jiang JK, Lake JP, et al. The manegement of complicated diverticulitis and the role of computed tomography. The American Journal of Gastroenterology. 2005;**100**:910-917

[9] Nascimbeni R, Amato A, Cirocchin R, Serventi A, Laghi A, Bellini M, et al. Management of perforated diverticulitis with generalized peritonitis. A multidisciplinary review and position paper. Techniques in Coloproctology. 2021;**25**:153-165

[10] Rafferty J, Shellito P, Hyman NH, Buie WD. Standards Committee os American Society of Colon and Rectal Surgeons Practice parameters for sigmoid diverticulitis. Diseases of the Colon and Rectum. 2006;**49**(7):939-944

[11] Siewart B, Tye G, Kruskal J, Sosna J, Opelka F. Impact of CT-guided drainage in the treatment of diverticular abscesses: Size matters. American Journal of Roentgenology. 2006;**186**:680-686

[12] Amborsetti P, Chautems R, Soravia C, Peiris-Waser N, Terrier F. Long-term outcome of mesocoic and pelvic diverticular abscesses of the left colon: A prospective study of 73 cases. Diseases of the Colon and Rectum. 2005;**48**(4):787-791

[13] Fowler H, Gachabayov M, Vimalachandran D, Clifford R, Orangio GR, Bergamaschi R. Failure of nonoperative management in patients with acute diverticulitis complicated by abscess: A systematic review. International Journal of Colorectal Disease. 2021;**36**:1367-1383

[14] Garfinkle R, Kugler A, Pelsser V, Vasilevsky C-A, Morin N, Gordon P, et al. Diverticular abscess managed with long-term definitive nonoperative intent is safe. Diseases of the Colon and Rectum. 2016;**59**(7):648-655

[15] Biffoni M, Urciuoli P, Grimaldi G, Eberspacher C, Santoro A, Pironi D, et al. Colovesical fistula complicating diverticular disease: Diagnosis and

surgical management in elderly. Minerva Chirurgica. 2019;**74**:187-8

[16] Strati TM, Sapalidis K, Koimtzis GD, Pavlidis E, Atmatzidis S, Liavas L, et al. Sigmoido-cecal fistula: A rare case of complicated recurrent diverticulitis and a review of the literature. American Journal of Case Reports. 2018;**19**: 1386-1392

[17] Badic B, Leroux G, Thereaux J, Joumond A, Gancel CH, Bail JP, et al. Colovesical fistula complicating diverticular disease: A 14-year experience. Surgical Laparoscopy, Endoscopy & Percutaneous Techniques. 2017;**27**(2):94-97

[18] Maciel V, Lujan HJ, Plasencia G, et al. Diverticular disease complicated with colovesical fistula: Laparoscopic versus robotic management. International Surgery. 2014;**99**:203-210

[19] Bertelson NL, Abcarian H, Kalkbrenner KA, Blumetti J, Harrison JL, Chaundhry V, et al. Techniques in Coloproctology. 2018;**22**:31-36

[20] El-Haddad HM, Kassem MI, Sabry AA, Abouelfotouh A. Surgical protocol and outcome for sigmoidovesical fistula secondary to diverticular disease of the left colon: A retrospective cohort study. International Journal of Surgery. 2018;**56**:115-123

[21] Cavalcanti NS et al. Infecção do trato urinário de repetição por fistula enterovesical secundária a doença diverticular do colon: um relato de caso. Jornal Brasileiro de Nefrologia. 2013;**35**(4):341-345

[22] Reis LDO, Rodrigues M, Reis C, Mendes L, Cardoso-Filho C, Costa A, et al. Sigmoidovesical fistula complicating diverticular disease: Report of six cases. Relato de casos Cirurgia. 2021;7(3):e2654. DOI: 10.30928/2527-2039e-20212654

[23] Mendez-Pastor A, Garcia-Henriquez N. Complicated diverticulitis. Diseases of the Colon and Rectum. 2020;**63**:26-29

[24] Golabek T, Szymanska A, Szopinski T, et al. Enterovesical fistulae: Aetiology, imaging and management. Gastroenterology Research and Practice. 2013;**2013**:617967

[25] Marney L, Ho YH. Laparoscopic management of diverticular colovesical fistula: Experience in 15 cases and review of the literature. International Surgery. 2013;**98**:101-109

[26] Boselli C, Gemini A, Cirocchi R, Grassi V, Avenia S, Polistena A, et al. It is safe and useful, laparoscopic peritoneal lavage in the treatment of acute diverticulitis of octogenarian patients? A multicenter retrospective observational study. Aging Clinical and Experimental Research. 2017; **29**(Suppl 1):83-89

[27] Reis LDOR, Lombardi OA, Reis ADO, Cardoso EH, Cardoso Filho CAM. Cirurgia de Hartmann – Analise de 41 casos em hospital de referência no Norte do Paraná. Revista Brasileira de Coloproctologia. 2001;**21**(1):19-22

[28] Park JS, Choi G-S, Park SI, et al. Randomised clinical trial of robot assisted versus standard laparoscopic right colectomy. The British Journal of Surgery. 2012;**99**:1219-1226

[29] Dolejs AJ, Penning AJ, Gusmann MJ, Fajardo AD, Holcomb BK, Robb BW, et al. Perioperative manegement of patients with colovesical fistula. Journal of Gastrointestinal Surgery. 2019;**23**: 1867-1873

[30] Tancer ML, Veridiano NP. Genital fistulas caused by diverticular disease of the sigmoid colon. American Journal of Obstetrics and Gynecology. 1996;**174**(5): 1547-50

[31] Berger MB, Khandwala N, Fenner DE, Burney RE. Colovaginal fistulas – Presentation, evaluation and management. Female Pelvic Medicine and Reconstructive Surgery. 2016;**22**(5): 355-358

[32] Siegle JC, Glasgow JÁ, Chatfield RB. Late sequelae of histerectomy and diverticulosis: Colovaginal fistulae. The Journal of the Oklahoma State Medical Association. 1992;**85**(6):227-80

[33] Hain JM, Sherik DG, Cleary RK. Salpingocolonic fistula secundar to diverticulitis. The American Surgeon. 1996;**62**(12):984-6

[34] Lisbon E, Bloom RA, Verstanding A, Lax E, Lutwak E. Sigmoid-apendiceal fistula in diverticular disease. Diagnostic Imaging in Clinical Medicine. 1984;**53**(5):262-4

[35] Safatle NF, Filardi CG, Almeida MC, Ciasca Junior DV, Saflate AM. Sigmoidovaginal fistulas. Report of 3 cases. São Paulo Medical Journal. 1986;**104**(4):221-3

[36] VanBuren WM, Lightner AM, Kim ST, Sheedy SP, Wooleyer MC, Menias CO, et al. Imaging and surgical management of anorectal vaginal fistulas. Radiographics. 2018;**38**:13851401

[37] Dessole L, Capobianco E, Noya G, Meloni GB. Interposition of fallopian salpinges in the treatment of sigmoidvaginal fistula, secondary to vaginal histerectomy with failure of previous repair. Archives of Gynecology and Obstetrics. 2000;**264**(1):45-46

[38] Yashi M, Muraishi O, Yuzawa M, Tokue A. A case of colo-vesico-vaginal fistula caused by sigmoid colon diverticulitis. Hinyokika Kiyo. 1998;**44**(7):513-5

[39] Vasilevsky CA, Belliveau P, Trudel JL, Stein BL, Gordon PH. Fistulas complicating diverticulitis. International Journal of Colorectal Disease. 1998;**13**(2):57-60

[40] Hjern F, Goldberg SM, Johansson C, Parker SC, Mellgren A. Management of diverticular fistulae to the female genital tract. Colorectal Disease. 2007;**9**(5): 438-42

[41] Khalaf C, Houlind KC. Case report: Primary aortosigmoid fistula – A rare cause of lower gastrointestinal bleeding. International Journal of Surgery Case Reports. 2017

[42] Reis LDO, Moreira RCR. Fistula aorto-sigmoideana primária - relato de um caso. Rev bras Colo-Proct 1989;**9**(3): 113-115

Section 4

Antibiotics in Diverticulitis

Chapter 5

The Use of Antibiotics in Diverticulitis: An Update in Non-operative Management

Mariana Morales-Cruz and Paulina Moctezuma Velázquez

"Antibiotics prescription was considered the standard procedure for an episode of acute noncomplicated diverticulitis; nowadays, in well-selected patients, antibiotics may be avoided."

Abstract

Diverticulosis is a common disease among Western and developed nations. Approximately 20% of patients with diverticulosis will become symptomatic. Acute diverticulitis is a common manifestation of diverticular disease. Different classifications exist to try to categorize it but, it is generally considered as complicated or uncomplicated. Eighty-five percent of patients with an acute onset of diverticulitis will have an uncomplicated presentation. The best way to assess the degree and severity of the disease is a CT scan along with some biochemical parameters like CRP. Recent guidelines from associations all over the world accept non-antibiotic therapy as a valid strategy of treatment for the non-complicated diverticulitis. Antibiotics are still compulsory in immune-compromised patients, the elderly, those with comorbidities, and those with signs of sepsis. Recommendations should be made on a case-by-case basis.

Keywords: uncomplicated diverticulitis, outpatient treatment, antibiotics, conservative management

1. Introduction

Diverticulosis is a common disease among the Western and developed nations; its prevalence increases with age, being 10% in adults over 40 years and around 70% in patients over 80 years. Approximately 20% of patients with diverticulosis will become symptomatic [1].

Worldwide, the incidence of diverticular disease is rising. Lifestyle and Western diet seem to be the factors influencing this epidemiological change, increasing most dramatically among age groups between 18 and 64 years old. Amid young patients, diverticular disease is more common in men, while in the elderly population, the prevalence is similar between both sexes [2]. Diverticular disease can occur in any part of the colon, but the left side is more frequently affected in Western countries, while up to 70% of cases in Asia appear on the right side [3].

Different classifications exist to categorize acute diverticulitis, but it is generally classified as uncomplicated or complicated. The computed tomography of the abdomen and pelvis is the best way to assess its severity. Further investigations to characterize it include white blood cell count and C-reactive protein levels [4]. About 85% of patients that attend to the emergency department for an acute onset of diverticular disease will have an uncomplicated form of it, and they may be treated conservatively [5]. The rest of the cases will present with abscess, fistula, perforation, stricture, or peritonitis, where surgical treatment is advised in an urgent or elective setting. Surgical options are diverse, but the indications and recommendations to choose one strategy over the other are beyond the scope of this chapter.

Regarding nonoperative management, patients can be hospitalized or sent home with or without antibiotics. Treatment should be tailored according to the patient's characteristics [6]. Patients with uncomplicated diverticulitis by CT may develop severe complications in 1.4% of the cases [7], while recurrence rates have been described to be from 5 to 20% [8]. Recurrence risk tends to be higher in patients with a previous episode of complicated diverticulitis (24% vs. 23.4%, $p = 0.622$) rather than in patients with uncomplicated diverticulitis, and most of these episodes occur within the first year [9] of the initial onset.

2. Discussion

2.1 Medical approach of uncomplicated diverticulitis

Diverticulitis treatment has been modified throughout time. The prescription of antibiotics used to be the therapeutic foundation of it, but it could be avoided now in well-selected patients [10]. The nonantibiotic treatment strategy was formulated more than a decade ago when diverticular physiopathology was reassessed. At first, it was known that diverticular occlusion, micro-perforation, and peritoneal infection were the origin of diverticulitis [11]. Later, with the finding of TNF-a overexpression, it was concluded that inflammation plays a crucial role in diverticulitis development [12]. Even more, patients with diverticular disease seem to have changed in the gastrointestinal flora, including the depletion of some fecal microbiota species that have anti-inflammatory properties [13]. Subjects with diverticula seem to have more macrophages in the intestinal wall than their healthier counterparts, promoting inflammation rather than infection [14] and therefore raising the question about the actual need for antibiotics for its treatment during an acute flare.

Under this hypothesis, anti-inflammatory medication has been suggested as a treatment for acute uncomplicated diverticulitis, spearing the use of antibiotics as long as complications are not present.

Two of the most important contributions regarding the avoidance of the use of antibiotics were made by the AVOD (Antibiotika Vid Okomplicerad Divertikulit—Swedish for "antibiotics in uncomplicated diverticulitis") and DIABOLO (DIverticulitis: AntiBiotics Or cLose Observation?) randomized control trials (RCT), published in 2011 and 2016, respectively.

The DIABOLO study [15] was a multicentric trial evaluating two different approaches for the management of uncomplicated acute diverticulitis, either observation or antibiotic treatment. The patients included were those with the first episode of left-sided uncomplicated diverticulitis, classified according to Hinchey's or Ambrosetti's scale. The diagnosis was confirmed with a CT scan in the first 24 h of presentation.

The antibiotic used was amoxicillin-clavulanic acid (unless allergic), and it was handed intravenously four times a day for the first 2 days and then switched to oral three times a day until a 10-day course was completed. For the initial doses, all the patients had to be admitted contrary to the observational group, which was treated in the outpatient setting as long as the patient could tolerate a regular diet, there was no fever, and there was reasonable pain control. Only 34 patients were sent home under this premise.

The primary analyses included 528 patients. The median time to recovery during 6 months follow-up was 14 days for patients who had conservative management vs. 12 days among those with antibiotics. Readmission rates were comparable: 17.6% in the observation vs. 12.0% in the antibiotic group ($p = 0.148$).

The proportion of patients with recurrent diverticulitis was similar in the two groups (3.4 vs. 3.0%; $p = 0.494$). Rates of sigmoid resection were comparable (3.8 vs. 2.3%; $p = 0.323$) for both emergency resection (0.8 vs. 1.1%; $p = 0.553$) and elective resection (3.1 vs. 1.1%; $p = 0.254$). In both groups, the most common reason for sigmoid resection was colonic obstruction (3 of 10 in the observation group vs. 2 of 6 in the antibiotic group), followed by perforation (2 of 10 vs. 2 of 6).

Another multicenter trial was the AVOD [7], where 10 surgical departments in Sweden and one in Iceland participated. Uncomplicated diverticulitis was defined as an episode of clinical signs compatible with diverticulitis, including fever and raised inflammatory markers complemented with computed tomography (CT). The randomization was done with sealed envelopes, and the patients were treated with just intravenous fluids or with antibiotic therapy, but in any case, hospital admission was required. A total of 623 patients were enrolled in the study—309 patients in the no-antibiotics arm and 314 in the antibiotics group. In the antibiotics group, the treatment was initiated with an intravenous combination of a cephalosporin (cefuroxime or cefotaxime) and metronidazole, or with carbapenem antibiotics or piperacillin-tazobactam, and then changed to an oral regimen for completion of 7 days. The discharge was made after the improvement of clinical and biochemical parameters in both groups. Further investigations with colonoscopy, barium enema, or CT colonography were made if none of these were performed within 1 year before admission at 6 or 8 weeks. No significant differences were found between patients treated with or without antibiotics. Neither did between the frequencies in surgery, length of hospital stay, recurrence of diverticulitis, chronic pain, or changes in bowel habit after 12 months.

This study group recently published a long-term follow-up of this cohort. At a median time of 11 years, the authors found no significant differences between the two groups in terms of recurrences (both 31.3%), complications, surgery for diverticulitis, or reported quality of life (EQ-5DTM) [16].

It is extremely important to mention that both trials supporting the avoidance of antibiotics included only patients with early-stage disease (Hinchey I and Ia). These RCTs are also prone to perform a selection bias because no blinding was made, and actual rates among centers were variable. Antibiotic treatment was also not standardized [17].

van Dijk et al. [18] made an individual-patient data meta-analysis with 1109 patients of the DIABOLO and AVOD trials: 545 in the observational group and 564 in the antibiotics group. To make results comparable, he redefined some of the concepts evaluated—ongoing diverticulitis, recurrent diverticulitis, and complicated diverticulitis. Ongoing diverticulitis was the persistence of symptoms during the following 3 months after initial discharge, and recurrent diverticulitis was defined as any episode occurring after discharge. The mean duration of follow-up was 12 months. Baseline characteristics were similar among groups; however, primary diverticulitis was slightly and significantly more common in the antibiotics group 454 cases vs. 408 in the nonantibiotic ($p = 0.029$). The length of stay for the initial hospital admission was shorter, although nonsignificant in the observational group. The rate of ongoing diverticulitis was 7.2% (39 of 545) in the observational group vs. 5.0% (28 of 564) in the antibiotics group ($p = 0.062$). The rates of recurrent diverticulitis were comparable: 8.6% (47 of 545) vs. 9.6% (54 of 564), respectively ($p = 0.610$). The rate of complicated diverticulitis within 1 month was 1.8% (10 of 545) in the observational group vs. 1.1% (6 of 564) in the antibiotics group ($p = 0.204$); at 1-year follow-up, it was 4% (22 of 545) vs. 2.1% (12 of 564), respectively ($p = 0.079$). Rates of sigmoid resection were no differences between the groups at 1 month or 1 year.

Other studies with less statistical power (non RCT) have had the same findings as to the DIABOLO and AVOD. Some meta-analyses have been made trying to gather more evidence about this topic, and the main outcomes address the recurrence, need for surgery, complication rate, and treatment failure.

A meta-analysis from Desai et al. [19], with seven studies for a total of 2241 patients, concluded that recurrent diverticulitis was actually slightly higher among patients who received antibiotics compared with those who did not 12.6% vs. 11.5% [pooled rate of recurrent diverticulitis OR = 1.27 (95%, CI = 0.90–1.79); $p = 0.18$]. Total complications were higher among patients who had antibiotics 27.8% vs. 19.85% [pooled OR = 1.99 (95% CI, 0.66–6.01); $p = 0.22$), and so was treatment failure 3% vs. 4.5% (pooled OR = 0.68 (95% CI, 0.42–1.09); $p = 0.11$], and readmission rates 14.5% vs. 15.2% [pooled OR = 0.75 (95% CI, 0.44–1.30); $p = 0.31$], pointing out that all negative outcomes tend to be lower in the nonantibiotic group, although no statistical significance was found in any of them. But it is also worth mentioning that the rate of sigmoidectomy was higher in the patients treated without antibiotics, 1.5% vs. 4.8% [pooled OR = 3.37 (95% CI, 0.65–17.34); $p = 0.15$]. In the end, the benefit of treating patients without antibiotics was proven in fewer costs, less hospital stays, and less antibiotic resistance.

Emile et al. [20] published a systematic review of nine studies with 2565 patients. Failure was defined as the deterioration of symptoms requiring an antibiotic prescription or the readmission within 1 month of discharge due to persistency of them, with or without complications. Recurrence was defined as a new episode of diverticulitis within 1 month after discharge, and readmission was defined as a hospital admission within 1 year after discharge. They concluded that there were no differences in treatment failure, (OR = 1.5, $p = 0.06$), recurrence (OR = 0.81, $p = 0.2$), complications rate (OR = 0.56, $p = 0.25$), hospital readmissions (OR = 0.97, $p = 0.91$), need for surgery (OR = 0.59, $p = 0.28$), or mortality (OR = 0.64, $p = 0.47$). In this meta-analysis, the only predictor for failure in the nonantibiotic group was associated comorbidities ($p < 0.001$). Other authors found that a CRP higher than 170 mg/dL was also associated with treatment failure.

A Cochrane systematic review from 2012 [21], including three randomized control trials, found no difference in outcomes between patients with uncomplicated diverticulitis treated with or without antibiotics. The patients included in the analyzed studies were healthy with a Hinchey I or Ia stage of the disease.

Mege and Yeo [22] made a meta-analysis including 2321 patients from 11 different studies. The primary endpoint was treatment failure, recognizing this as the need for emergency surgery (0.7% vs. 1.4%; $p = 0.1$). The secondary outcome was a recurrence, this being readmission for a new episode of acute diverticulitis 1 month after the previous episode (11% vs. 12%; $p = 0.3$). Then again, no difference was found. Emergency surgery occurred less frequently in the observational group than in the treatment group (0.5% vs. 1%, $p = 0.34$), and even elective surgery happened at comparable rates. But if we consider only the randomized control trials included, elective surgery occurred in 0.9% of the patients treated with antibiotics vs. 2.5% in the antibiotic group ($p = 0.04$).

The reason why elective surgery may be more frequently performed in patients in the nonantibiotic group might be the misperception of being undertreated, so they sought a definitive treatment. Antibiotics may reduce low-grade colonic inflammation avoiding complications such as obstruction, recurrence, or ongoing diverticulitis [11].

Another meta-analysis included nine studies; two RCT, five cohort studies, and two case-control studies, with a total of 1164 patients. In this, patients treated without antibiotics required an additional intervention or treatment in 5.3% of the cases vs. the 3.6% on the antibiotic group but without statistical significance (risk ratio = 1.48; p = 0.28) [17]. The study concluded that treatment without antibiotics is associated with a shorter hospital stay and no difference in readmission rates (risk ratio = 1.17; p = 0.26), need for surgical or radiological intervention (risk ratio = 0.61; p = 0.34), recurrence (risk ratio = 0.83; p = 0.21), and complications (risk ratio = 0.70–1.18; p = 0.67–0.91).

Mocanu et al. [23] performed another meta-analysis considering two RCT, one single-center cohort, two retrospective cohorts, one prospective cohort, one retrospective case control, and one prospective cohort single arm with a total of 2469 patients. The outcomes included were—recurrence (readmission greater than 1 month following intervention), treatment failure (recurrence of symptoms within 1 month of intervention), abscess, bleeding, fistula, perforation, stenosis, and need for elective or emergent surgery. The overall complication rate was 18.7%, and there was no difference among groups 17.7% in the nonantibiotic group vs. 20.2% in the antibiotic group (OR = 0.72; CI = 0.45–1.16; p = 0.18). Recurrence was the most common seeing with a rate between 2 and 28%. The rates of abscesses, perforation, stenosis, elective and emergency surgery were also no different. There was a statistical difference in the length of stay being 1 day less for the nonantibiotic group. They concluded that antibiotic use in patients with acute uncomplicated diverticulitis is not associated with a reduction in significant complications.

Daniels et al. [24] ran a pragmatic RCT with the analysis of the information from 528 patients. His observational strategy proved no inferiority when compared to the antibiotic treatment for the first episode of uncomplicated diverticulitis. The duration of initial admission was longer, and the rate of antibiotic-related adverse events was higher in the antibiotic group, suggesting that antibiotics can be omitted. He also mentions that 7.3% of the patients treated without antibiotics had ongoing diverticulitis vs. 4.7% in the antibiotic group p = 0.183.

Quality of life between both treatments has not been adequately addressed; there is a lack of information regarding this critical outcome. Ongoing diverticulitis might not be a precise indicator of the quality of life, but it does make reference to the persistency of symptoms, which may affect the quality of life of patients [24].

The number of days, type of antibiotics, and inpatient or outpatient administration are the other questions arousing in regard to uncomplicated diverticulitis treatment. Antibiotic therapy must be effective against aerobic (*Escherichia coli*, *Proteus*, *Klebsiella*, and *Enterococcus*) and anaerobic (*Bacteroides*, *Clostridium*, *Bifidobacterium*, and *Peptostreptococcus*) bacteria. In general, a broad-spectrum antibiotic should be elected or combination therapy with metronidazole and quinolones or third-generation cephalosporins or beta-lactam antibiotics with a beta-lactamase inhibitor [10]. Under the premise of reducing antibiotic resistance and costs, Schug-Pass et al. [25] designed a randomized trial to elucidate whether short-term therapy (4 days) with ertapenem is as effective as standard therapy (7 days) in an inpatient scenario. Randomization was conducted on day 4, with antibiotic therapy being then either terminated or continued for a further three days. In uncomplicated sigmoid diverticulitis, symptomatic improvement happens in the first 96 h. This prospective randomized trial demonstrated that a shorter 4-day treatment period is just as effective as the standard treatment (98.0% vs. 98.2%).

A prospective, single-arm study overviewed [26] the safety and efficacy of symptomatic (nonantibiotic) treatment for CT-proven uncomplicated acute diverticulitis during a 30-day follow-up period. A total of 153 patients (95%) completed the follow-up. A total of 14 (9%) patients had pericolic gas. Altogether, 140 (87%) patients were treated as outpatients, and four (3%) of them were admitted to the hospital at some point. The primary outcome of this study was to find the progression to complicated diverticulitis. None of the subjects developed it or needed surgery, but 2 days (median) after inclusion, antibiotics were given to 14 (9%, six orally, eight intravenously) patients.

Jackson and Hammond [27] did a systematic review back in 2014 justified by the lack of evidence to support the traditional inpatient treatment with bowel rest, intravenous fluids, and intravenous antibiotics. This review included nine studies (415 patients) where all, except for one, used either CT scan or US to confirm uncomplicated diverticulitis. Once the diagnosis was made, some protocols would discharge patients immediately on oral antibiotics and a liquid diet for 10 days. Other protocols would keep patients in the hospital for 24 h before sending them home. Three of the studies allowed some patients to have outpatient care even with abscesses between 2 and 3 cm. About 403 patients out of a total of 415 (97%) participants were successfully treated in the outpatient setting, concluding that a more progressive, ambulatory-based approach is effective and safe.

Another systematic review including 21 studies (11 prospectives, nine retrospectives, and only one randomized trial) with 1781 patients was recently published by Cirocchi et al. [28]. Outpatient management for acute left diverticulitis was the primary outcome evaluated. The meta-analysis concluded that outpatient management is safe. The overall failure rate was 4.3% (95% CI = 2.6–6.3%). Ambulatory treatment was associated with an estimated daily cost savings of between €600 and €1900 per patient treated.

With the growing evidence that antibiotic therapy is not essential for the treatment of acute uncomplicated diverticulitis, several guidelines support the observational management in afebrile clinically stable cases.

A survey conducted in 2011 [29] between gastroenterologists and surgeons found a general opinion about antibiotics not being for everyone any longer. The Danish and Dutch guidelines from 2011 to 2012, respectively, do not recommend the routine use of antibiotics [30].

The American Gastroenterological Association in 2015 advised that antibiotics should be used selectively rather than routinely in patients [31]. Stating also that treatment with broad-spectrum antibiotics may not solve the symptomatology in patients with acute uncomplicated diverticulitis. However, antibiotics may decrease the risk of recurrence and diverticular complications in comparison with no antibiotics. The effect of antibiotics on the development of sepsis and the need for surgery or colostomy remains uncertain.

Recent guidelines from associations all over the world now consider nonantibiotic therapy as a valid strategy for uncomplicated acute diverticulitis, among this associations the American Society of Colorectal Surgeons Clinical practice guidelines for the treatment of left-sided colonic diverticulitis (2020) [32], the Second International Symposium on Diverticular Disease [33], held in Rome in 2016, and the 2020 WSES guidelines [34] address that CT scan findings must be compatible with uncomplicated acute diverticulitis and patients must not show signs of sepsis. The WSES established that immunocompetent patients with uncomplicated diverticulitis without signs of systemic inflammation should not receive antibiotic therapy. This was supported too by last year's ESCP guidelines [35]; the commissioning guide for colonic diverticular disease made by the Royal College of Surgeons of England [36] in 2014, and the Japanese Gastroenterological Association [37] in 2019.

The EAES and SAGES [38] guidelines also make a remark about the immunocompetence of the patients, establishing those healthy individuals with uncomplicated acute diverticulitis will have similar outcomes with just symptomatic treatment. The antibiotic prescription should be reserved for immunocompromised patients and cases with sepsis. The recommendations from other societies can be found in **Table 1**.

Society	Recommendation	Grade of evidence	References
World Society of Emergency Surgery (WSES): update of the guidelines for the management of acute colonic diverticulitis in the emergency setting (2020)	In immunocompetent patients with uncomplicated diverticulitis without signs of systemic inflammation, we recommend not to prescribe antibiotic therapy	1A	Cochrane Review, AVOD, Mali et al., DIABOLO and DIABOLO LONG TERM
American Society of Colon and Rectal Surgeons (ASCRS): clinical practice guidelines for the treatment of left-sided colonic diverticulitis (2020)	Selected patients with uncomplicated diverticulitis can be treated without antibiotics	1A	AVOD, DIABOLO, Mege et al., Sánchez-Velázquez: systematic review, Isacson et al., Van Dijk ST, COCHRANE, Estrada Ferrer et al., Desai et al., Au S et al., Emile et al. Mocanu et al., Bolkenstein
European Society of Coloproctology (ESCP): Guidelines for the management of diverticular disease of the colon (2020)	Patients with acute uncomplicated diverticulitis do not require antibiotics routinely. Antibiotic treatment should be reserved for immunocompromised patients and patients with sepsis	Strong	AVOD, Isacson et al., van Dijk ST et al., Desai M et al., Daniels L et al.
EAES and SAGES 2018 consensus conference on acute diverticulitis management: evidence-based recommendations for clinical practice	In immunocompetent individuals presenting with uncomplicated acute diverticulitis, symptomatic treatment without antibiotics provides similar outcomes to treatment with antibiotics	Weak	Galetin T et al., Kohler L et al.
American Gastroenterological Association Institute Guideline on the Management of Acute Diverticulitis	Antibiotics should be used selectively rather than routinely in acute uncomplicated diverticulitis	Low quality	AVOD, DIABOLO, Stollman AGA, Sultan S AGA, Graham et al., Peery AF, Feingold D, et al., Morris et al.
American Gastroenterological Association Institute Technical Review on the Management of Acute Diverticulitis (2015)	Treatment with broad-spectrum antibiotics for at least seven days may not improve symptom resolution. Nevertheless, it may decrease the risk of recurrence and diverticular complications	Low quality	COCHRANE, Morris AM et al., DIABOLO, Daniels LUC, de Korte N A et al., Hjern F et al.

Society	Recommendation	Grade of evidence	References
Guidelines of Diagnostics and Treatment of Acute Left-Sided Colonic Diverticulitis (Netherlands)	Antibiotic treatment is recommended when signs of generalized infection and affected general condition or signs of bacteremia or septicemia are present. Antibiotic treatment is recommended in immunocompromised patients	Level A2	Ridgway PF et al., AVOD Schug-Pass C et al.
Danish national guidelines for the treatment of diverticular disease	The use of antibiotics in uncomplicated diverticulitis is justified by septicemia, affected general condition, pregnancy, or immuno-suppression. Antibiotics are not routinely recommended	Ib	Kaiser et al., Sarin S, Chautems et al., Schug-Pass C et al., Byrnes MC et al., AVOD , Hjern F et al
Italian Society of Colon and Rectal Surgery. Practice parameters for the treatment of colonic diverticular disease: Guidelines	The suggestion of avoiding antibiotics in acute uncomplicated diverticulitis may not improve short- or long-term outcomes. Use only on a case-by-case basis	Ib	AVOD, Andersen JC, et al., Westwood DA et al., Hjern F et al., DIABOLO
Diverticular disease: guidelines of the German Society for Gastroenterology, Digestive and Metabolic Diseases and the German Society for General and Visceral Surgery	In acute uncomplicated left-sided diverticulitis with no risk indicators for a challenging course, antibiotic therapy can be omitted subject to close clinical monitoring	Open recommendations	AVOD, Hjern F et al., Schug-Pass C et al.
Royal College of Surgeons (RCS) of England: Commissioning guide—Colonic diverticular disease (2014)	There is low-level evidence that patients suitable for management at home may be managed without the use of antibiotics		COCHRANE
Japan Gastroenterological Association (JGA): Guidelines for colonic diverticular bleeding and colonic diverticulitis (2019)	Antibiotic therapy has been reported to be unnecessary for colonic diverticulitis without abscess or perforation, but no studies have been conducted in Japan. Therefore, the efficacy of antibiotic therapy among Japanese patients is currently unclear. Antibiotic therapy is considered acceptable in current clinical practice	C	Brochmann ND et al., AVOD, DIABOLO, Isacson D et al., Daniels L et al.

Table 1.
Recommendations on the treatment of noncomplicated acute left diverticulitis.

2.2 Right-sided colonic uncomplicated diverticulitis.

Right-sided diverticulosis is a rare condition in the Western population, but it is often seen in Asian countries. Its prevalence does not increase with age as it happens with the sigmoid diverticula. Right colon diverticula are usually solitary, true (all layers), and congenital; muscle hypertrophy is not observed [39]. Acute right diverticulitis episodes generally occur in middle-aged men [40]. Differential diagnosis is complex, and it is frequently misinterpreted as acute appendicitis. There is not much literature regarding the treatment for right-sided diverticulitis.

The only study we were able to find about this subject was the one made by Destek and Gül [41] with 22 patients. Nine (40.9%) were female, and 13 (59%) were male. The age range was 26–84 years, with a mean age of 50.9 years. The duration of symptoms (nausea, diarrhea, and pain) prior to hospitalization was 1–5 days. In general, leukocytosis was detected in 77.2% of all patients, and high CRP levels were found in all of them (100%). About 59% of the patients had diverticulitis in the right colon, and 41% of them had diverticulitis in the cecum. Patients were classified as Hinchey stage I or II. Symptomatic conservative treatment was applied in 19 patients (86.3%). Oral intake was discontinued for 2 or 3 days, intravenous hydration therapy with balanced solutions was given, intravenous dual antibiotic therapy was applied, and after 2–8 days, they were discharged with oral regimes. A percutaneous drainage catheter was placed under sonography in four patients (18.1%) in whom the localized abscess did not regress with conservative treatment.

Generally speaking, most recent guidelines support the use of the same principles already discussed for the treatment of right-sided diverticulitis.

2.3 Uncomplicated diverticulitis and diet

For years, patients have been instructed to consume a clear-liquid or low-residue diet (low fiber), or even to deprive themselves of food for bowel rest during the diverticulitis flare [42, 43]. Several guidelines have supported this. A survey conducted in the Netherlands in 2011 showed that 83.2% of participating gastroenterologists and surgeons advised some form of bowel rest [42], but the Dutch guideline of 2012 stated that an unrestricted diet could also be advised [44].

In the prospective, observational study published by Isacson et al. [45] in 2015, patients with confirming CT scan for uncomplicated diverticulitis were enrolled to receive recommendations on oral intake of fluids for the first 48 h followed by a liquid diet and then moving on to a complete diet as tolerated. Readmission within 1 month with or without complications was defined as a management failure. In total, 155 patients were included in the study, and only four patients had treatment failure. Five patients (3.3%) had a recurrence within the 3-month follow-up period.

A prospective, uncontrolled study of an unrestricted diet in 86 patients with uncomplicated diverticulitis concluded that this was well tolerated, although 8% had serious adverse events and 20% had ongoing symptoms [46].

A high-dietary fiber diet is hypothesized to prevent diverticulitis reoccurrence by reducing the contact time between stool and diverticula [47]. There has been an increased in the use of probiotic supplementation under the assumption of them decreasing the risk of infection and inflammation of the diverticula [48].

The systematic review of Dahl et al. [49] addressed the lack of high-quality reports and research about the dietary management of adults with acute, uncomplicated diverticulitis. However, generalized observations tended to agree that either a free diet or a restricted one is equal in terms of recovery. A multicenter trial is underway to evaluate an unrestricted vs. a progressive diet in uncomplicated diverticulitis.

3. Conclusions

The nonantibiotic management in patients with uncomplicated diverticulitis still has some unsettled topics like management of the right-sided or recurrent uncomplicated disease; further investigation in different populations and world regions is needed. More supervision on antibiotic prescription needs to be encouraged in patients who receive therapy for acute diverticulitis to make a cost-effect analysis for each case [50].

In conclusion, antibiotics may not improve outcomes in acute uncomplicated diverticulitis, but the high mortality associated with sepsis requires clinicians to maintain a low threshold in high-risk individuals such as immunocompromised patients, the elderly, and those with comorbidities [51]. Therefore, recommendations should be made on a case-by-case basis. If antibiotic therapy is necessary, oral administration is equally as effective as intravenous administration, and an expeditious switch from intravenous to oral may allow the fastest patient discharge.

Conflict of interests

Authors declare no conflict of interests.

Author details

Mariana Morales-Cruz[1]* and Paulina Moctezuma Velázquez[2]

1 Department of Colorectal Surgery, Queen Elizabeth Hospital, Birmingham, UK

2 Hospital ABC, Ciudad de México, Mexico

*Address all correspondence to: marmocru@gmail.com

References

[1] Hanna MH, Kaiser AM. Update on the management of sigmoid diverticulitis. World Journal of Gastroenterology. 2021;**27**(9):760-781. DOI: 10.3748/wjg.v27.i9.760

[2] Hawkins AT, Wise PE, Chan T, Lee JT, Glyn T, Wood V, et al. Diverticulitis: An update from the age-old paradigm. Current Problems in Surgery. 2020;**57**(10):100862. DOI: 10.1016/j.cpsurg.2020.100862. Epub 2020 Jul 18

[3] Weizman AV, Nguyen GC. Diverticular disease: Epidemiology and management. Canadian Journal of Gastroenterology. 2011;**25**(7):385-389. DOI: 10.1155/2011/795241

[4] O'Leary DP, Lynch N, Clancy C, Winter DC, Myers E. International, expert-based, consensus statement regarding the management of acute diverticulitis. JAMA Surgery. 2015;**150**(9):899-904. DOI: 10.1001/jamasurg.2015.1675

[5] Masoomi H, Buchberg BS, Magno C, Mills SD, Stamos MJ. Trends in diverticulitis management in the United States from 2002 to 2007. Archives of Surgery. 2011;**146**(4):400-406. DOI: 10.1001/archsurg.2010.276

[6] Shahedi K, Fuller G, Bolus R, et al. Long-term risk of acute diverticulitis among patients with incidental diverticulosis found during colonoscopy. Clin Gastroenterol Hepatol. Dec 2013;**11**(12):1609-13. DOI: 10.1016/j.cgh.2013.06.020. Epub 2013 Jul 12. PMID: 23856358; PMCID: PMC5731451

[7] Chabok A, Påhlman L, Hjern F, Haapaniemi S, Smedh K, AVOD Study Group. Randomized clinical trial of antibiotics in acute uncomplicated diverticulitis. The British Journal of Surgery. 2012;**99**(4):532-539. DOI: 10.1002/bjs.8688. Epub 2012 Jan 30

[8] Feingold D, Steele SR, Lee S, Kaiser A, Boushey R, Buie WD, et al. Practice parameters for the treatment of sigmoid diverticulitis. Diseases of the Colon & Rectum. 2014;**57**(3):284-294. DOI: 10.1097/DCR.0000000000000075

[9] Eglinton T, Nguyen T, Raniga S, Dixon L, Dobbs B, Frizelle FA. Patterns of recurrence in patients with acute diverticulitis. The British Journal of Surgery. 2010;**97**(6):952-957. DOI: 10.1002/bjs.7035

[10] Jacobs DO. Clinical practice. Diverticulitis. New England Journal of Medicine. 2007;**357**(20):2057-2066. DOI: 10.1056/NEJMcp073228

[11] Peery AF, Sandler RS. Diverticular disease: Reconsidering conventional wisdom. Clinical Gastroenterology and Hepatology. 2013;**11**(12):1532-1537. DOI: 10.1016/j.cgh.2013.04.048

[12] Tursi A, Scarpignato C, Strate LL, Lanas A, Kruis W, Lahat A, et al. Colonic diverticular disease. Nature Reviews Disease Primers. 2020;**6**(1):20. DOI: 10.1038/s41572-020-0153-5. Erratum in: Nat Rev Dis Primers. 2020 Apr 29;**6**(1):35. Erratum in: Nat Rev Dis Primers. 2020 Jun 17;6(1):50

[13] Barbara G, Scaioli E, Barbaro MR, et al. Gut microbiota, metabolome and immune signatures in patients with uncomplicated diverticular disease. Gut. 2017;**66**:1252-1261

[14] Floch MH, White JA. Management of diverticular disease is changing. World Journal of Gastroenterology. 2006;**12**(20):3225-3228. DOI: 10.3748/wjg.v12.i20.3225

[15] Unlü C, de Korte N, Daniels L, Consten EC, Cuesta MA, Gerhards MF, et al. A multicenter randomized clinical trial investigating the cost-effectiveness of treatment strategies with or without

antibiotics for uncomplicated acute diverticulitis (DIABOLO trial). BMC Surgery. 2010;**10**:23. DOI: 10.1186/1471-2482-10-23

[16] Isacson D, Smedh K, Nikberg M, Chabok A. Long-term follow-up of the AVOD randomized trial of antibiotic avoidance in uncomplicated diverticulitis. The British Journal of Surgery. 2019;**106**(11):1542-1548. DOI: 10.1002/bjs.11239. Epub 2019 Aug 6

[17] Au S, Aly EH. Treatment of uncomplicated acute diverticulitis without antibiotics: A systematic review and meta-analysis. Diseases of the Colon & Rectum. 2019;**62**(12): 1533-1547. DOI: 10.1097/ DCR.0000000000001330

[18] van Dijk ST, Chabok A, Dijkgraaf MG, Boermeester MA, Smith K. Observational *versus* antibiotic treatment for uncomplicated diverticulitis: An individual patient data meta-analysis. British Journal of Surgery. 2020;**107**(8):1062-1069. DOI: 10.1002/bjs.11465

[19] Desai M, Fathallah J, Nutalapati V, Saligram S. Antibiotics versus no antibiotics for acute uncomplicated diverticulitis: A systematic review and meta-analysis. Diseases of the Colon and Rectum. 2019;**62**(8): 1005-1012. DOI: 10.1097/DCR. 0000000000001324

[20] Emile SH, Elfeki H, Sakr A, Shalaby M. Management of acute uncomplicated diverticulitis without antibiotics: A systematic review, meta-analysis, and meta-regression of predictors of treatment failure. Techniques in Coloproctology. 2018;**22**(7):499-509. DOI: 10.1007/ s10151-018-1817-y Epub 2018 Jul 6

[21] Shabanzadeh DM, Wille-Jørgensen P. Antibiotics for uncomplicated diverticulitis. Cochrane Database of Systematic Reviews. 2012;(11) Art. No.: CD009092 10.1002/14651858.CD009092.pub2

[22] Mege D, Yeo H. Meta-analyses of current strategies to treat uncomplicated diverticulitis. Diseases of the Colon and Rectum. 2019;**62**(3):371-378. DOI: 10.1097/DCR.0000000000001295

[23] Mocanu V, Dang JT, Switzer N, Tavakoli I, Tian C, de Gara C, et al. The role of antibiotics in acute uncomplicated diverticulitis: A systematic review and meta-analysis. American Journal of Surgery. 2018;**216**(3):604-609. DOI: 10.1016/j. amjsurg.2018.01.039. Epub 2018 Feb 2

[24] Daniels L, Ünlü Ç, de Korte N, van Dieren S, Stockmann HB, Vrouenraets BC, et al. Randomized clinical trial of observational *versus* antibiotic treatment for a first episode of CT-proven uncomplicated acute diverticulitis. British Journal of Surgery. 2017;**104**(1):52-61. DOI: 10.1002/ bjs.10309

[25] Schug-Pass C, Geers P, Hügel O, Lippert H, Köckerling F. Prospective randomized trial comparing short-term antibiotic therapy versus standard therapy for acute uncomplicated sigmoid diverticulitis. International Journal of Colorectal Disease. 2010;**25**(6):751-759. DOI: 10.1007/ s00384-010-0899-4. Epub 2010 Feb 6. Erratum in: Int J Colorectal Dis. 2010 Jun;25(6):785

[26] Mali JP, Mentula PJ, Leppäniemi AK, Sallinen VJ. Symptomatic treatment for uncomplicated acute diverticulitis: A prospective cohort study. Diseases of the Colon and Rectum. 2016;**59**:529-534

[27] Jackson JD, Hammond T. Systematic review: Outpatient management of acute uncomplicated diverticulitis. International Journal of Colorectal Disease. 2014;**29**:775-781

[28] Cirocchi R, Randolph JJ, Binda GA, Gioia S, Henry BM, Tomaszewski KA, et al. Is the outpatient management of acute diverticulitis safe and effective? A systematic review and meta-analysis. Techniques in Coloproctology. 2019;**23**(2):87-100. DOI: 10.1007/s10151-018-1919-6. Epub 2019 Jan 25

[29] de Korte N, Unlü C, Boermeester MA, Cuesta MA, Vrouenreats BC, Stockmann HB. Use of antibiotics in uncomplicated diverticulitis. The British Journal of Surgery. 2011;**98**(6):761-767. DOI: 10.1002/bjs.7376. Epub 2011 Jan 6

[30] Vennix S, Morton DG, Hahnloser D, Lange JF, Bemelman WA, Research Committee of the European Society of Coloproctology. Systematic review of evidence and consensus on diverticulitis: An analysis of national and international guidelines. Colorectal Disease. 2014;**16**(11):866-878. DOI: 10.1111/codi.12659

[31] Stollman N, Smalley W, Hirano I, AGA Institute Clinical Guidelines Committee. American Gastroenterological Association Institute guideline on the management of acute. Diverticulitis. Gastroenterology. 2015;**149**(7):1944-1949. Epub 2015 Oct 8. DOI: 10.1053/j.gastro.2015.10.003

[32] Hall J, Hardiman K, Lee S, Lightner A, Stocchi L, Paquette IM, et al. The American Society of colon and rectal surgeons clinical practice guidelines for the treatment of left-sided colonic diverticulitis. Diseases of the Colon and Rectum. 2020;**63**(6): 728-747. DOI: 10.1097/DCR.0000000000001679

[33] Tursi A, Picchio M, Elisei W, Di Mario F, Scarpignato C, Brandimarte G. Management of patients with diverticulosis and diverticular disease: consensus statements from the 2nd International Symposium on Diverticular Disease. Journal of Clinical Gastroenterology. 2016;**50**(Suppl 1):S101-S107. DOI: 10.1097/MCG.0000000000000654

[34] Sartelli M, Weber DG, Kluger Y, et al. 2020 update of the WSES guidelines for the management of acute colonic diverticulitis in the emergency setting. World Journal of Emergency Surgery: WJES. 2020;**15**:32. DOI: 10.1186/s13017-020-00313-4

[35] Schultz JK, Azhar N, Binda GA, Barbara G, Biondo S, Boermeester MA, et al. European Society of Coloproctology: Guidelines for the management of diverticular disease of the colon. Colorectal Disease. 2020;**22**(Suppl 2):5-28. DOI: 10.1111/codi.15140. Epub 2020 Jul 7

[36] Available from: https://www.rcseng.ac.uk/library-and-publications/rcs-publications/docs/colinic-diverticular-disease/

[37] Nagata N, Ishii N, Manabe N, Tomizawa K, Urita Y, Funabiki T, et al. Guidelines for colonic diverticular bleeding and colonic diverticulitis: Japan gastroenterological association. Digestion. 2019;**99**(Suppl 1):1-26. DOI: 10.1159/000495282. Epub 2019 Jan 9

[38] Francis NK, Sylla P, Abou-Khalil M, Arolfo S, Berler D, Curtis NJ, et al. EAES and SAGES 2018 consensus conference on acute diverticulitis management: evidence-based recommendations for clinical practice. Surgical Endoscopy. 2019;**33**(9):2726-2741. DOI: 10.1007/s00464-019-06882-z. Epub 2019 Jun 27

[39] Radhi JM, Ramsay JA, Boutross-Tadross O. Diverticular disease of the right colon. BMC Research Notes. 2011;**4**:383

[40] Stollman N, Raskin JB. Diverticular disease of the colon. Lancet. 2004;**363**: 631-639

[41] Destek S, Gül VO. Effectiveness of conservative approach in right colon diverticulitis. Ulusal Travma ve Acil Cerrahi Dergisi. 2019;**25**:396-402

[42] Korte N, Klarenbeek B, Kuyvenhoven J, et al. Management of diverticulitis: Results of a survey among gastroenterologists and surgeons. Colorectal Disease. 2011;**13**:e411-e417

[43] Rafferty J, Shellito P, Hyman NH, Buie WD. Standards committee of American Society of colon and rectal surgeons practice parameters for sigmoid diverticulitis. Diseases of the Colon and Rectum. 2006;**49**:939-944. DOI: 10.1007/s10350-006-0578-2

[44] Andeweg CS, Felt-Bersma R, Verbon A, Stoker J, Boermeester M, Bleichrodt R. Summary of the practice guideline on diverticulitis in the colon: diagnostics and treatment in specialty care. Nederlands Tijdschrift voor Geneeskunde. 2013;**157**(15):A6124

[45] Isacson D, Thorisson A, Andreasson K, Nikberg M, Smith K, Chabok A. Outpatient, non-antibiotic management in acute uncomplicated diverticulitis: A prospective study. International Journal of Colorectal Disease. 2015;**30**(9):1229-1234. DOI: 10.1007/s00384-015-2258-y. Epub 2015 May 20. Erratum in: Int J Colorectal Dis. 2015 Sep;30(9):1235

[46] Stam MA, Draaisma WA, van de Wall BJ, et al. An unrestricted diet for uncomplicated diverticulitis is safe: results of a prospective diverticulitis diet study. Colorectal Disease. 2017;**19**:372

[47] Commane DM, Arasaradnam RP, Mills S, Mathers JC, Bradburn M. Diet, ageing and genetic factors in the pathogenesis of diverticular disease. World Journal of Gastroenterology. 2009;**15**:2479-2488. DOI: 10.3748/wjg.15.2479

[48] Tursi A, Brandimarte G, Giorgetti GM, Elisei W, Aiello F. Balsalazide and/or high-potency probiotic mixture (VSL# 3) in maintaining remission after attack of acute, uncomplicated diverticulitis of the colon. International Journal of Colorectal Disease. 2007;**22**:1103-1108

[49] Dahl C, Crichton M, Jenkins J, et al. Evidence for dietary fibre modification in the recovery and prevention of reoccurrence of acute, uncomplicated diverticulitis: A systematic literature review. Nutrients. 2018;**10**(2):137. DOI: 10.3390/nu10020137

[50] Huston JM, Zuckerbraun BS, Moore LJ, Sanders JM, Duane TM. Antibiotics versus no antibiotics for the treatment of acute uncomplicated diverticulitis: Review of the evidence and future directions. Surgical Infections. 2018;**19**(7):648-654. DOI: 10.1089/sur.2018.115. Epub 2018 Sep 11

[51] Sartelli M, Viale P, Catena F, Ansaloni L, Moore E, Malangoni M, et al. 2013 WSES guidelines for management of intra-abdominal infections. World Journal of Emergency Surgery: WJES. 2013;**8**:3

Section 5

Colonoscopy in Diverticulitis

Chapter 6

Colonoscopy after Diverticulitis

Jeremy Meyer and Frédéric Ris

Abstract

Patients suffering from diverticulitis are at increased risk for colorectal cancer and should undergo colonoscopy to rule out colorectal cancer. The prevalence of colorectal cancer in this population was estimated to range between 1.9 and 2.3%. This prevalence is higher in patients with complicated diverticulitis (abscess, perforation) and ranges between 6.1% and 7.9%. Therefore, interval colonoscopy is strongly recommended after an episode of complicated diverticulitis. The prevalence of colorectal cancer is lower in patients with uncomplicated diverticulitis and approaches the prevalence from screened populations. In patients with uncomplicated diverticulitis, the indication for colonoscopy is still a matter of debate and should be done on a case-by-case basis.

Keywords: Colonoscopy, endoscopy, sigmoidoscopy, diverticulitis, diverticular disease, colorectal cancer

1. Introduction

Diverticulitis is defined as the inflammation of a diverticulum confirmed by imaging and associated with compatible clinical presentation and laboratory tests [1].

First imaging modalities for diverticulitis included plain film radiography of the abdomen, contrast enema and abdominal ultrasound. However, due to their low sensitivity and specificity for the diagnosis of diverticulitis, these imaging techniques became quickly supplanted by computed tomography (CT). CT features of acute diverticulitis consist in signs of local inflammation [2], such as thickening of the colonic wall close to the diverticulum, peri-diverticulum and/or peri-colonic fat stranding and, in case of perforation, peri-colonic or distant air bubbles, pericolonic abscess, pelvic fluid or extra-colonic feces.

Several classifications systems have been developed based on CT findings [3, 4], such as the Neff classification [5], the Kaiser classification [6] and the Hansen-Stock [7] classification. However, the most commonly used classification system is the hybrid score (both radiological and clinical) of Hinchey modified by Wasvary [8]. Classification of diverticulitis tailors its therapeutic management. More commonly, diverticulitis is usually classified into uncomplicated diverticulitis and complicated diverticulitis [1]. Uncomplicated diverticulitis is defined as the local inflammation of a diverticulum (and its associated segment of bowel) without any sign of perforation and/or abscess (corresponding to modified Hinchey 1a [8]), whereas complicated diverticulitis is defined as an acute diverticulitis with a covered perforation [9–12] (Hansen-Stock I/IIa [7]), with a paracolic abscess (modified Hinchey

1b [8]), with a distant abscess (Hinchey II [8]), or with a purulent (Hinchey III [8]) or fecal peritonitis (Hinchey IV [8]).

According to the Global Burden of Disease Study, the number of incident cases of colorectal cancer (CRC) was of 1.8 million for year 2017, with a 9.5% increase in the age-standardized incidence rate within 30 years. Moreover, CRC accounted for 896,000 deaths and 19 million disability-adjusted life-years in 2017 [13]. As a consequence, several countries have implemented screening programs, either with fecal tests and/or with colonoscopy, which allowed reducing the incidence of CRC (by removing polyps) and the mortality related to CRC (by early detection of CRC) [14]. Despite these public health interventions, CRC is often still discovered by CT protocolled to investigate weight loss, iron-deficiency anemia, change in bowel habits and/or abdominal pain. If suspicion for CRC is raised on CT, flexible sigmoidoscopy or colonoscopy are requested to confirm the diagnosis with biopsies, tattoo the lesion for potential surgery and rule out any additional synchronous CRC.

However, in patients presenting with abdominal pain and/or sepsis in the acute setting, interpretation of the CT becomes more difficult, especially in the presence of diverticular disease, whose prevalence is increasing with aging. For the radiologist and for the surgeon, distinguishing with certitude between diverticulitis and CRC is not always possible, as both pathologies share similar imaging features of local and/or distant inflammation [15–17].

Considering the difficulty in ruling out CRC based solely on CT in patients initially diagnosed with diverticulitis, recommendations have emerged in favor of interval colonoscopy after diverticulitis.

2. Colonoscopy in patients with diverticular disease

The incidence of CRC was found to be increased by 5.8-fold in patients with diverticular disease when compared to reference patients without diverticular disease [18]. However, this risk was reported to be more important within the early period after diverticular disease-related hospitalization, before decreasing to the incidence of the reference population after 2 years [19, 20]. Therefore, it is likely that the increased risk of CRC observed in the short-term follow-up period reflects initial misdiagnosis of CRC as a diverticular disease-related complication (such as diverticulitis), rather than a true long-term risk for CRC. A systematic review and meta-analysis of cross-sectional studies (450,953 patients) found no association between diverticular disease and advanced colorectal neoplasia [21]. As a consequence, colonoscopy is currently not recommended in patients with uncomplicated diverticular disease, as this population is not at increased risk for CRC.

3. Colonoscopy after diverticulitis

The primary indication for performing colonoscopy after diverticulitis is to rule out CRC, with the rationale that patients with diverticulitis are at increased risk for CRC. Therefore, numerous observational studies have reported the prevalence and/or the incidence of CRC in patients diagnosed with diverticulitis, and were pooled into several systematic reviews with/without meta-analyses [22–27].

A recent and large systematic review and meta-analysis pooling both observational studies and population-based studies (50,445 patients) estimated the pooled prevalence of CRC to be of 1.9% in patients initially diagnosed with diverticulitis. This prevalence was of 2.3% when performing subgroup analysis including only studies based on colonoscopy. Moreover, the pooled prevalences of polyps, advanced adenomas and adenomas were estimated to be of 22.7%, 4.4% and 14.2%, respectively [25]. Another meta-analysis pooling only diverticulitis patients who underwent colonoscopy estimated the prevalence of CRC to be of 2.1%, and the prevalence of advanced colorectal neoplasia to be of 6.9% [24].

The incidence of CRC in diverticulitis patients is therefore higher than the incidence encountered in colonoscopy screening programs (which is approximately of 0.8% [28]). A recent observational study with a good sample size reported that patients with diverticulitis were at significantly higher risk (prevalence of 2.9%) for CRC than patients from a local colonoscopy register (prevalence of 0.3%) [29]. Moreover, patients who undergo colonoscopy are already considered at higher risk for CRC, as they were entered into the program due to either positive fecal test and/or red flags for CRC. The prevalence of CRC in this population may therefore be overestimated and not reflect the prevalence in the general population.

To ensure that patients suffering from diverticulitis are effectively at increased risk for CRC and should be targeted by endoscopic screening, the incidence of CRC in this population was compared to the incidence of CRC in a reference population, and was found to be 20 to 44-fold more important than in reference matched patients [30, 31].

Therefore, the current recommendation is that patients with diverticulitis should undergo colonoscopy to rule out CRC at least 6 weeks after the episode if no colonoscopy was done within the last 3 years. However, this recommendation differs depending on the severity of the diverticulitis episode [1].

4. Colonoscopy after uncomplicated diverticulitis

Uncomplicated diverticulitis is defined as diverticulitis without any evidence for abscess and/or perforation.

In this population, the prevalence of CRC was estimated to be of 1.3% by one large meta-analysis [25] and of 0.5% by a meta-analysis selectively including patients who underwent colonoscopy [24]. The prevalence of CRC in patients with uncomplicated diverticulitis is therefore low and close to the prevalence reported by colonoscopy screening programs (0.8% [28]). Of note, one study reported that the prevalence of CRC was of 1.2% in patients with uncomplicated diverticulitis versus 0.6% in patients from a CRC colonoscopy screening program, this difference not reaching significance [32]. Therefore, several authors have recommended to dispense patients with uncomplicated diverticulitis from colonoscopy. However, the interpretation of these data may be limited by the overestimation of the prevalence of CRC in patients from screening programs, which may not reflect the prevalence in the general population, and by heterogeneity of studies in the field.

Looking more specifically at studies which compared the incidence of CRC in patients with uncomplicated diverticulitis to the incidence of CRC in the general population, patients with uncomplicated episode may still constitute a population at risk for CRC. For instance, one study reported the incidence of CRC to be 40-fold higher in patients with uncomplicated diverticulitis than in age- and gender-matched reference patients, but was limited by a low number of incidental cases [31]. Another study documented an incidence that was 20-fold

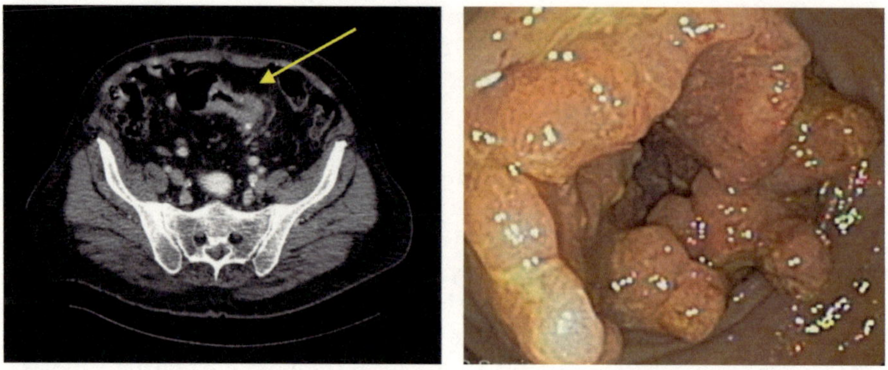

Figure 1.
Sixty-four year old female patient who presented with abdominal pain in the left iliac fossa and iron-deficiency anemia. Computed tomography reported an uncomplicated diverticulitis of the sigmoid colon (left, arrow). Flexible sigmoidoscopy found a suspect lesion at 23 cm from the anal verge (right), whose biopsies came back positive for an adenocarcinoma. The patient underwent a high anterior resection. Pathology of the operative specimen was pT3N2 (4/35).

higher in diverticulitis patients, but the study population was not limited to patients with uncomplicated diverticulitis and included all patients who had conservative management [30]. Finally, a population-based study cross-matched with data from the Cancer Registry of Norway estimated the standard morbidity ratio for CRC to be of 6.58 for patients with uncomplicated diverticulitis when compared to reference patients [33], therefore suggesting an increased risk in this population.

Moreover, colonoscopy carries a risk of complications [34]. For instance, the incidence of colonoscopy-related perforation was estimated to range between 0.09% [35] and 0.19% [36], and perforation was shown to significantly increase mortality when compared to patients without perforation [36]. Further, the cost per colonoscopy was recently evaluated to range between 188.6 USD and 501.2 USD (for purchase, maintenance and processing) [37, 38]. When considering that approximately 15 millions colonoscopies were performed in 2012 in the USA [39], targeting at risk populations is key to avoid increasing the costs for healthcare systems.

Considering the conflicting results regarding the prevalence of CRC in patients with uncomplicated diverticulitis, as well as the morbidity and cost of colonoscopy, the indication to perform colonoscopy after an episode of uncomplicated diverticulitis has remained controversial. Current guidelines recommend to do it on a case-by-case basis and to reserve it to symptomatic patients (**Figure 1**) [1, 40].

5. Colonoscopy after complicated diverticulitis

Complicated diverticulitis is by definition associated with abscess and/or perforation.

Radiological studies showed that abscess and perforation on CT are predictors for CRC [16, 22, 41–43]. Meta-analyses have estimated that the incidence of CRC in patients with complicated diverticulitis ranges between 6.1% [27] and 7.9% [25], and is 5–16.3 fold more important than in patients with uncomplicated diverticulitis [25, 27, 33].

Therefore, it is currently agreed that patients with complicated diverticulitis should undergo colonoscopy to rule out CRC (**Figure 2**) [1].

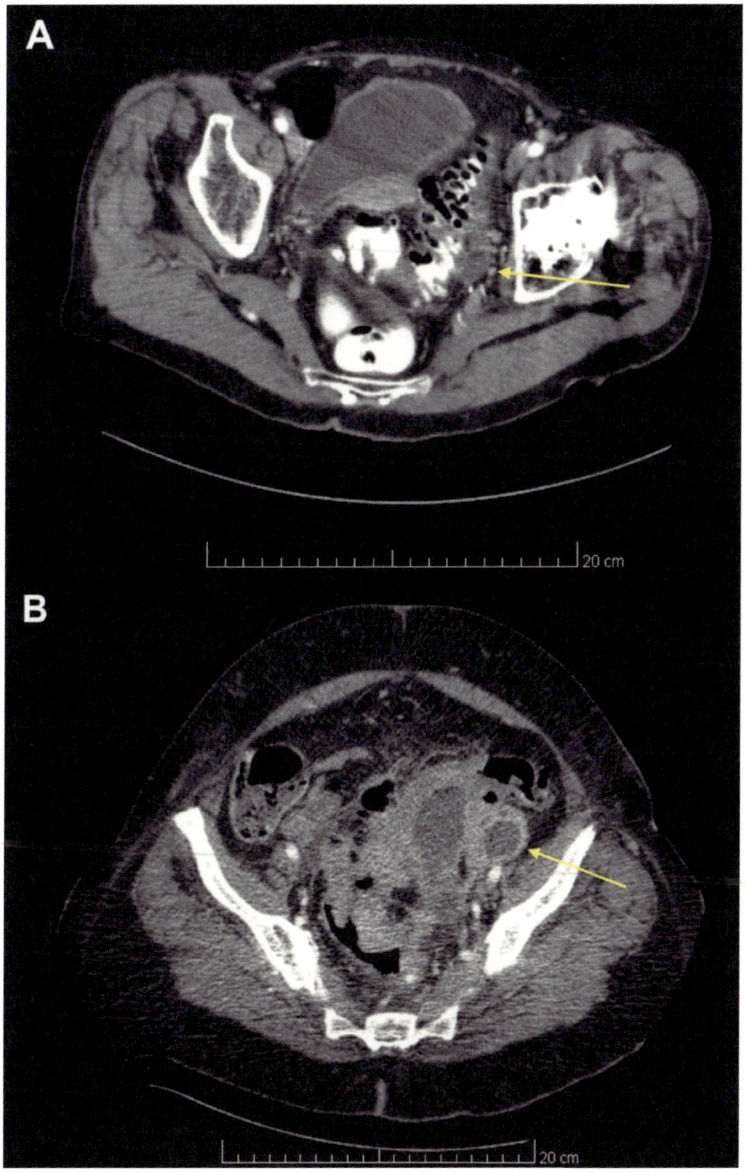

Figure 2.
(A) Ninety year old female patient who presented with acute abdominal pain in the left iliac fossa and localized guarding. Computed tomography showed a 3 cm paracolic abscess (arrow), and the episode was classified as Hinchey 1b. Due to poor response to conservative management, the patient underwent Hartmann procedure. Examination of the operative specimen found a pT1 N0 adenocarcinoma arising from a polyp close to the perforated diverticulum. (B) Eighty-five female patient who presented with lower abdominal pain. Computed tomography found a large paracolic abscess (arrows), and the episode was classified as Hinchey 1b. The patient underwent percutaneous drainage, which allowed to completely drain the abscess. However, interval computed tomography described an apple core imaging of the sigmoid. Flexible sigmoidoscopy found a lesion of the sigmoid compatible with cancer, and biopsies came back positive for adenocarcinoma. The patient underwent oncologic Hartmann, and pathology of the operative specimen came back as pT4 N1 (2/20).

6. Conclusion

Due to increased risk for CRC, colonoscopy should be performed after acute diverticulitis in patients with complicated episode or who remain symptomatic after uncomplicated episode.

Conflict of interest

The authors declare no conflict of interest.

Author details

Jeremy Meyer[1,2*] and Frédéric Ris[1,2]

1 University Hospitals of Geneva, Geneva, Switzerland

2 University of Geneva, Geneva, Switzerland

*Address all correspondence to: jeremy.meyer@hcuge.ch

References

[1] Schultz JK, Azhar N, Binda GA, et al. European Society of Coloproctology: guidelines for the management of diverticular disease of the colon. Colorectal Dis 2020;22 Suppl 2:5-28.

[2] Kircher MF, Rhea JT, Kihiczak D, et al. Frequency, sensitivity, and specificity of individual signs of diverticulitis on thin-section helical CT with colonic contrast material: experience with 312 cases. AJR Am J Roentgenol 2002;178: 1313-1318.

[3] Klarenbeek BR, de Korte N, van der Peet DL, et al. Review of current classifications for diverticular disease and a translation into clinical practice. Int J Colorectal Dis 2012;27:207-214.

[4] Feingold D, Steele SR, Lee S, et al. Practice parameters for the treatment of sigmoid diverticulitis. Dis Colon Rectum 2014;57:284-294.

[5] Neff CC, vanSonnenberg E. CT of diverticulitis. Diagnosis and treatment. Radiol Clin North Am 1989;27:743-752.

[6] Kaiser AM, Jiang JK, Lake JP, et al. The management of complicated diverticulitis and the role of computed tomography. Am J Gastroenterol 2005;100:910-917.

[7] Hansen O, Graupe F, Stock W. [Prognostic factors in perforating diverticulitis of the large intestine]. Chirurg 1998;69:443-449.

[8] Wasvary H, Turfah F, Kadro O, et al. Same hospitalization resection for acute diverticulitis. Am Surg 1999;65:632-635; discussion 636.

[9] Garcia-Gomez MA, Belmonte-Montes C, Cosme-Reyes C, et al. [Prognostic value of the presence of pericolic air bubbles detected by computed tomography in acute diverticulitis]. Cir Cir 2017;85:471-477.

[10] Bolkenstein HE, van Dijk ST, Consten ECJ, et al. Conservative Treatment in Diverticulitis Patients with Pericolic Extraluminal Air and the Role of Antibiotic Treatment. J Gastrointest Surg 2019.

[11] Mora Lopez L, Serra Pla S, Serra-Aracil X, et al. Application of a modified Neff classification to patients with uncomplicated diverticulitis. Colorectal Dis 2013;15:1442-1447.

[12] Meyer J, Caruso A, Roos E, et al. The clinical significance of extraluminal air in Hinchey 1a diverticulitis: results from a retrospective cohort study with 10-year follow-up. Int J Colorectal Dis 2019;34:2053-2058.

[13] Collaborators GBDCC. The global, regional, and national burden of colorectal cancer and its attributable risk factors in 195 countries and territories, 1990-2017: a systematic analysis for the Global Burden of Disease Study 2017. Lancet Gastroenterol Hepatol 2019;4:913-933.

[14] Cardoso R, Guo F, Heisser T, et al. Colorectal cancer incidence, mortality, and stage distribution in European countries in the colorectal cancer screening era: an international population-based study. Lancet Oncol 2021;22:1002-1013.

[15] Chintapalli KN, Chopra S, Ghiatas AA, et al. Diverticulitis versus colon cancer: differentiation with helical CT findings. Radiology 1999;210: 429-435.

[16] Balthazar EJ, Megibow A, Schinella RA, et al. Limitations in the CT diagnosis of acute diverticulitis: comparison of CT, contrast enema, and pathologic findings in 16 patients. AJR Am J Roentgenol 1990;154:281-285.

[17] Shen SH, Chen JD, Tiu CM, et al. Differentiating colonic diverticulitis

from colon cancer: the value of computed tomography in the emergency setting. J Chin Med Assoc 2005;68: 411-418.

[18] Stefansson T, Ekbom A, Sparen P, et al. Increased risk of left sided colon cancer in patients with diverticular disease. Gut 1993;34:499-502.

[19] Granlund J, Svensson T, Granath F, et al. Diverticular disease and the risk of colon cancer - a population-based case-control study. Aliment Pharmacol Ther 2011;34:675-681.

[20] Huang WY, Lin CC, Jen YM, et al. Association between colonic diverticular disease and colorectal cancer: a nationwide population-based study. Clin Gastroenterol Hepatol 2014;12: 1288-1294.

[21] Lee HJ, Park SJ, Cheon JH, et al. The relationship between diverticulosis and colorectal neoplasia: A meta-analysis. PLoS One 2019;14:e0216380.

[22] Sharma PV, Eglinton T, Hider P, et al. Systematic review and meta-analysis of the role of routine colonic evaluation after radiologically confirmed acute diverticulitis. Ann Surg 2014;259:263-272.

[23] Sai VF, Velayos F, Neuhaus J, et al. Colonoscopy after CT diagnosis of diverticulitis to exclude colon cancer: a systematic literature review. Radiology 2012;263:383-390.

[24] Rottier SJ, van Dijk ST, van Geloven AAW, et al. Meta-analysis of the role of colonoscopy after an episode of left-sided acute diverticulitis. Br J Surg 2019;106:988-997.

[25] Meyer J, Orci LA, Combescure C, et al. Risk of Colorectal Cancer in Patients With Acute Diverticulitis: A Systematic Review and Meta-analysis of Observational Studies. Clin Gastroenterol Hepatol 2019;17:1448-1456 e17.

[26] Daniels L, Unlu C, de Wijkerslooth TR, et al. Routine colonoscopy after left-sided acute uncomplicated diverticulitis: a systematic review. Gastrointest Endosc 2014;79:378-89; quiz 498-498 e5.

[27] Koo CH, Chang JHE, Syn NL, et al. Systematic Review and Meta-analysis on Colorectal Cancer Findings on Colonic Evaluation After CT-Confirmed Acute Diverticulitis. Dis Colon Rectum 2020;63:701-709.

[28] Niv Y, Hazazi R, Levi Z, et al. Screening colonoscopy for colorectal cancer in asymptomatic people: a meta-analysis. Dig Dis Sci 2008;53: 3049-3054.

[29] Tehranian S, Klinge M, Saul M, et al. Prevalence of colorectal cancer and advanced adenoma in patients with acute diverticulitis: implications for follow-up colonoscopy. Gastrointest Endosc 2020;91:634-640.

[30] Grahnat CJ, Herard S, Ackzell A, et al. High Probability of an Underlying Colorectal Cancer Among Patients Treated for Acute Diverticulitis. A Population-Based Cohort Follow-Up Study. World J Surg 2016;40:2283-2288.

[31] Meyer J, Thomopoulos T, Usel M, et al. The incidence of colon cancer among patients diagnosed with left colonic or sigmoid acute diverticulitis is higher than in the general population. Surg Endosc 2015;29:3331-3337.

[32] Daniels L, Unlu C, de Wijkerslooth TR, et al. Yield of colonoscopy after recent CT-proven uncomplicated acute diverticulitis: a comparative cohort study. Surg Endosc 2015;29:2605-2613.

[33] Azhar N, Buchwald P, Ansari HZ, et al. Risk of colorectal cancer following

CT-verified acute diverticulitis: a nationwide population-based cohort study. Colorectal Dis 2020;22:1406-1414.

[34] Kim SY, Kim HS, Park HJ. Adverse events related to colonoscopy: Global trends and future challenges. World J Gastroenterol 2019;25:190-204.

[35] Araghizadeh FY, Timmcke AE, Opelka FG, et al. Colonoscopic perforations. Dis Colon Rectum 2001;44:713-716.

[36] Gatto NM, Frucht H, Sundararajan V, et al. Risk of perforation after colonoscopy and sigmoidoscopy: a population-based study. J Natl Cancer Inst 2003;95:230-236.

[37] Larsen S, Kalloo A, Hutfless S. The hidden cost of colonoscopy including cost of reprocessing and infection rate: the implications for disposable colonoscopes. Gut 2020;69:197-200.

[38] Henry SG, Ness RM, Stiles RA, et al. A cost analysis of colonoscopy using microcosting and time-and-motion techniques. J Gen Intern Med 2007;22: 1415-1421.

[39] Joseph DA, Meester RG, Zauber AG, et al. Colorectal cancer screening: Estimated future colonoscopy need and current volume and capacity. Cancer 2016;122:2479-2486.

[40] Rottier SJ, van Dijk ST, Boermeester MA. Author response to Comment on: Meta-analysis of the role of colonoscopy after an episode of left-sided acute diverticulitis. Br J Surg 2020;107:154.

[41] Sallinen V, Mentula P, Leppaniemi A. Risk of colon cancer after computed tomography-diagnosed acute diverticulitis: is routine colonoscopy necessary? Surg Endosc 2014;28:961-966.

[42] Brar MS, Roxin G, Yaffe PB, et al. Colonoscopy following nonoperative management of uncomplicated diverticulitis may not be warranted. Dis Colon Rectum 2013;56:1259-1264.

[43] Lau KC, Spilsbury K, Farooque Y, et al. Is colonoscopy still mandatory after a CT diagnosis of left-sided diverticulitis: can colorectal cancer be confidently excluded? Dis Colon Rectum 2011;54:1265-1270.